O A E L

OXFORD AMERICAN ENDOCRINOLOGY LIBRARY

Type 1 Diabetes in Adults

O A E L
OXFORD AMERICAN ENDOCRINOLOGY LIBRARY

Type 1 Diabetes in Adults

Barbara Simon, MD
Chief, Division of Endocrinology
Assistant Professor of Medicine
Drexel University College of Medicine
Philadelphia, PA

Jeremy Flood, MD
Assistant Professor of Medicine
Drexel University College of Medicine
Philadelphia, PA

Serge Jabbour, MD
Associate Professor of Medicine
Interim Director, Division of Endocrinology
Thomas Jefferson University
Philadelphia, PA

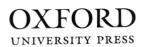

OXFORD
UNIVERSITY PRESS
2011

OXFORD
UNIVERSITY PRESS

Oxford University Press, Inc., publishes works that further
Oxford University's objective of excellence
in research, scholarship, and education.

Oxford New York

Auckland Cape Town Dar es Salaam Hong Kong Karachi
Kuala Lumpur Madrid Melbourne Mexico City Nairobi
New Delhi Shanghai Taipei Toronto

With offices in

Argentina Austria Brazil Chile Czech Republic France Greece
Guatemala Hungary Italy Japan Poland Portugal Singapore
South Korea Switzerland Thailand Turkey Ukraine Vietnam

Copyright © 2011 by Oxford University Press, Inc.

Published by Oxford University Press, Inc.
198 Madison Avenue, New York, New York 10016
www.oup.com

Oxford is a registered trademark of Oxford University Press

Library of Congress Cataloging-in-Publication Data
Simon, Barbara, M.D.
Type 1 diabetes in adults / by Barbara Simon, Jeremy Flood, Serge Jabbour.
   p. ; cm. — (Oxford American endocrinology library)
Includes bibliographical references.
ISBN 978-0-19-973780-2 (standard ed. : alk. paper)
1. Diabetes. I. Flood, Jeremy. II. Jabbour, Serge. III. Title. IV. Title: Type one diabetes in
adults. V. Series: Oxford American endocrinology library.
[DNLM: 1. Diabetes Mellitus, Type 1. WK 810 S594t 2010]
RC660.S566 2010
616.4′62–dc22   2009044428

Printed in the United States of America
on acid-free paper

Disclosures

Dr. Jabbour has served on the speakers bureaus for Amylin and Eli Lilly.

Contents

Introduction/Preface

At a time of dramatic increases in the prevalence of obesity, it is appropriate that type 2 diabetes has received a great deal of attention by the endocrinology community. Clearly, the management of insulin resistance and cardiovascular risk is a critical issue. However, it is important to also acknowledge and address type 1 diabetes, the prevalence of which is also increasing, and the management of which remains complex. Currently it is estimated that 10% to 15% of those with diabetes carry the diagnosis of type 1 diabetes, and frequently the diagnosis is not straightforward, as we recognize that more adults previously thought to have type 2 diabetes actually have late-onset type 1 diabetes (also termed latent autoimmune diabetes of the adult, or LADA). It is relatively more common in people who are white compared to people of African or Asian descent.

Over the past decade, tools for the management of type 1 diabetes have evolved so that we have the opportunity to more closely replicate normal physiologic insulin secretion with either basal-bolus insulin therapy or continuous subcutaneous insulin infusions. Besides insulin, we also have new therapies such as pramlintide. While these advances allow us to better manage our patients with type 1 diabetes, they also add complexity. There have also been advances in the understanding of how type 1 develops, and new research in prevention strategies. This text addresses the concepts behind the care of the person with type 1 diabetes for endocrinologists and primary care providers.

Chapter 1

Diagnosis, Pathophysiology, and Prediction

Definition and Diagnosis

Type 1A diabetes mellitus (autoimmune diabetes) is characterized by auto-immune destruction of beta cells resulting in loss of insulin production, and dependence on insulin administration. Type 1B (idiopathic) diabetes mellitus results from non-autoimmune destruction of beta cells, and evidence of auto-immunity cannot be demonstrated.

Type 1A diabetes typically presents with acute symptomatic hyperglycemia and diabetic ketoacidosis. The dramatic presentation of ketoacidosis is more typical in younger patients. In adults, type 1 may also present with ketoacidosis, but it can also present with classic symptoms of hyperglycemia (polyuria, poly-dipsia, polyphagia, weight loss) or even asymptomatically with a mild degree of hyperglycemia or prediabetes (such as in LADA, see p. 7).

All types of diabetes mellitus are diagnosed by blood glucose level. According to the 2009 American Diabetes Association Standards of Care,[1] a random blood glucose level ≥200 mg/dL with signs and symptoms of diabetes, a fasting blood glucose of ≥126 mg/dL, or a glucose of ≥200 mg/dL after an oral glucose toler-ance test all make the diagnosis of diabetes mellitus (Table 1.1).

Hemoglobin A1c has been discussed as a method to diagnose diabetes in nonpregnant individuals. An expert panel of the American Diabetes Association recommends that an A1c value of 6.5% or greater should be used for the diagnosis of diabetes.[2] The A1c test may be more useful in diagnosing type 2 diabetes mellitus, with its chronic hyperglycemia usually not characterized by absolute insulin deficiency. The panel specifically mentions that type 1 diabetes, with its usual classic clinical onset in children and adolescents, should continue to be diagnosed clinically, and that A1c testing can be used in the absence of specific clinical conditions. As typical type 1A diabetes usually presents with an acute onset of hyperglycemia, the A1c may not reflect the current acute hyperglycemia. Caution must be used in interpreting the A1c level, which may have limitations in certain settings, such as the presence of blood loss, transfu-sion, hemoglobinopathies, and age-related increases.[2] Furthermore, in adults, a mild elevation in A1c may sway healthcare providers to make an assumption of type 2 diabetes and attempt treatment with an oral hypoglycemic medica-tion, rather than recognizing the features of type 1 or LADA and the need for insulin treatment. We recommend using the blood glucose value paired with

Table 1.1 Criteria for the Diagnosis of Diabetes

FPG ≥126 mg/dL (7.0 mmol/L). Fasting is defined as no caloric intake for at least 8 h*

OR

Symptoms of hyperglycemia and a casual plasma glucose ≥200 mg/dL (11.1 mmol/L). Casual is defined as any time of day without regard to time since last meal. The classic symptoms of hyperglycemia include polyuria, polydipsia, and unexplained weight loss.

OR

2-h plasma glucose ≥200 mg/dL (11.1 mmol/L) during an OGTT. The test should be performed as described by the World Health Organization, using a glucose load containing the equivalent of 75 g anhydrous glucose dissolved in water.*

*In the absence of unequivocal hyperglycemia, these criteria should be confirmed by repeat testing on a different day.
FPG = Fasting Plasma Glucose, OGTT = Oral Glucose Tolerance Test.
From: American Diabetes Association. Diagnosis and classification of diabetes mellitus. *Diabetes Care.* 2009;32:S66.

the examination of clinical features and antibody testing (see p. 8) to make the diagnosis of type 1 diabetes in adults.

Pathophysiology

Genetics, the environment, and possibly other unknown factors contribute to the development of type 1 diabetes. It is believed that an environmental trigger incites an autoimmune attack on the beta cells in persons who are genetically susceptible. Most evidence indicates that the immune response results from an imbalance of pathogenic and regulatory T lymphocytes,[3] with resulting destruction of the beta cells, and formation of antibodies to beta-cell antigens. The autoimmune destruction of the beta cells may take months or years, at which time markers of autoimmunity can be demonstrated but clinical diabetes has not yet developed.

More is being learned about genetic susceptibility. The risk for developing type 1 is increased in close relatives; risk is approximately 6% for offspring and 5% in siblings, with a concordance rate of 5% for fraternal (dizygotic) twins, and an increased concordance rate of 30% to 50% in identical (monozygotic) twins.[4] Genes within the MHC (HLA complex) region of chromosome 6p21 confer the greatest risk of developing disease; the majority of these genes encode antigen-presenting molecules.[5] The DR3/DR4 alleles in this region increase the risk; they are present in approximately 90% of patients with autoimmune type 1 diabetes (the HLA DR3-DQ2/DR4-DQ8 genotype is the highest-risk genotype). However, the HLA DQB1 0602 allele may confer protection against the development of type 1; it is present in less than 1% of children with diabetes.[6] There are also non-MHC genes that may affect susceptibility to type 1, though they may contribute only modestly to disease risk.[5] Polymorphisms found in the promoter regions of the insulin gene, a lymphocyte-specific tyrosine phosphatase gene, and cytotoxic T-lymphocyte-associated antigen gene have all been associated with an increased risk of type 1.[7,8]

While the inciting environmental trigger to the immunologic response is still unclear, multiple theories and agents have been postulated. The hygiene hypothesis proposes that improved sanitation and reduction of childhood illnesses increase the incidence of immune-mediated disorders.[9] Viral infections (coxsackievirus and enteroviruses) and vaccinations have also been investigated, but data are far from conclusive. Dietary factors such as early exposure to cow's milk have also been debated; however, prospective studies have not confirmed a link,[10] and the issue may be compounded by the fact that vitamin D (in fortified milk) may protect against the development of type 1.[11]

Autoimmunity

Once the autoimmune attack is triggered, antibodies to antigens within the beta cells can be detected in the serum. Insulin antibodies are usually the first to appear, followed by other islet cell antibodies (ICAs). Antibodies to the islet enzyme glutamic acid decarboxylase (GAD, or GAD 65) are found in approximately 70% of patients with type 1 at the time of diagnosis, and antibodies to the protein tyrosine phosphatase, insulinoma-associated protein 2 (IA-2), in 58% of patients with type 1.[12] One or both antibodies (GAD 65 and IA-2) are present in 90% of patients with new-onset type 1A diabetes.[13]

ICAs have been detected in rare syndromes that are associated with type 1 diabetes, which have helped in the understanding of the pathogenesis and autoimmune nature of type 1. Approximately 20% of patients with autoimmune polyendocrine syndrome type 1 (APS1) develop type 1 diabetes.[14] This condition results from mutation in the autoimmune regulator (AIRE) gene, which controls expression of autoreactive T lymphocytes, and is defined by the presence of two out of the three conditions of mucocutaneous candidiasis, adrenal insufficiency, and hypoparathyroidism. IPEX (immune dysregulation, polyendocrinopathy, enteropathy, X-linked) is a rare syndrome that causes overwhelming autoimmunity in neonates (including diabetes) and results from a mutation in a transcription factor controlling the development of regulatory T cells. Twenty to 50% of patients with autoimmune poylendocrine syndrome type 2 (APS2) have type 1 diabetes[15]; this syndrome is associated with autoimmune thyroid disease and adrenal insufficiency.

Type 1 diabetes is also associated with other autoimmune conditions, such as thyroid disease, vitiligo, Addison's disease, celiac disease, pernicious anemia, and autoimmune hepatitis. Approximately 15% to 30% of patients with type 1 diabetes have autoimmune thyroid disease (hypothyroidism being the most common), 4% to 9% have celiac disease, and 0.5% have Addison's disease (adrenal insufficiency).[14] These conditions are associated with their organ-specific antibodies (thyroid peroxidase, tissue transglutaminase, and 21-hydroxylase antibodies respectively), and screening for these conditions at the time of diagnosis of type 1 diabetes is recommended in the appropriate clinical setting, with periodic screening thereafter if clinical suspicion arises. Patients should be screened for thyroid disease every 1 to 2 years with a TSH level; more frequent testing is recommended for those with positive thyroid antibodies. In patients with positive adrenal antibodies, periodic screening for symptoms and ACTH stimulation testing should be performed. In those without adrenal antibodies, screening should be repeated if clinical findings occur. Adults with type 1 diabetes should be evaluated for symptoms of celiac disease, with further testing as clinically warranted.

Prediction

As mentioned, those with high-risk HLA genotypes have an approximately 6% lifetime risk of developing type 1 diabetes compared to those without,[16] and first-degree relatives of patients with type 1 have an increased risk of developing disease compared to the general population. While certain genotypes are predictive for the development of type 1 diabetes, the presence of antibodies to islet cell molecules in a high titer can also identify those at risk.[17]

In the period before the development of overt diabetes, detection of insulin autoantibodies, ICA, GAD, and IA-2, is possible. In offspring of parents with type 1 diabetes, children who develop antibodies early (before age 2) and develop multiple autoantibodies tend to progress to type 1 diabetes at a young age (in childhood).[18] A positive test for two out of three islet autoantibodies is highly predictive of progression to type 1 diabetes[3] in both relatives of type 1 patients and those in the general population. Higher titers of antibodies may also confer more risk.[19]

In the preclinical period before development of overt diabetes, measurement of an abnormal first-phase insulin response to glucose with intravenous or oral glucose tolerance testing in high-risk individuals is also predictive.[20] In patients with positive autoantibodies, an impairment of the first-phase insulin response on intravenous glucose tolerance testing gives a projected 5-year risk of type 1 of greater than 50%.[21]

Although there is no way to prevent type 1 diabetes, there is a significant interest in prediction of disease, particularly in families of patients with type 1. High-risk HLA genotyping, while predictive in first-degree relatives, would have a relative low yield in the general population, given the relatively high prevalence of these genotypes in Caucasian populations and the respective prevalence of type 1 diabetes in the general population. A better strategy may be to start with autoantibody detection, with GAD and IA-2 antibody testing. If positive, then secondary testing for additional autoantibodies (islet cell and insulin antibodies) can be performed.[22] If antibodies are positively identified, genotyping can be performed for further investigation and for evaluation of eligibility into ongoing prevention research trials.

Latent Autoimmune Diabetes of Adulthood (LADA)

While classic type 1A diabetes can present in adulthood, there is another subset of the adult population who typically present with milder hyperglycemia, similar to type 2 diabetes, yet they typically have a poor response to oral hypoglycemic agents and progress to insulin deficiency. This form of diabetes, termed LADA, is characterized by its diagnosis in adulthood, eventual insulin deficiency, and evidence of immune destruction of beta cells (patients have positive autoantibodies). It is also described as a slowly progressing type 1 diabetes and has also been labeled as "type 1.5 diabetes."

Among newly diagnosed diabetic adults thought to have type 2 diabetes, approximately 10% have LADA.[23] Like classic type 1 diabetes, there are genetic factors and likely environmental contributors that lead to beta cell destruction; however, the pathophysiology of LADA is less studied that in type 1A diabetes. There are no twin studies in LADA, but there is less twin concordance for development of type 1 diabetes if it occurs after age 25 (6%).[24] LADA patients do have high rates of HLA DR3 and DR4 alleles and demonstrate ICA positivity.[25]

In type 1 diabetes, often more than one antibody to the islet cells is present, whereas in LADA, it is more common to find single antibody positivity. It is more common to find ICAs and GAD in LADA, and less common to detect IA-2 and insulin autoantibodies.[26] It appears that progression to overt diabetes in antibody-positive patients is much faster at younger ages and slower in adulthood. In the Diabetes Prevention Trial (DPT),[27] relatives of patients with type 1 who had positive antibodies were evaluated for the presence of diabetes. The patients with prediabetes, or impaired glucose tolerance, as opposed to overt diabetes, were older (mean age 21). This characteristic slower progression of beta-cell destruction in LADA may occur because of a less pronounced genetic predisposition, possible protective genes, the development of immune tolerance, or possible varying exposure to environmental triggers.[25]

The rate of progression to dependence on insulin varies. Some patients progress within months; others may take years. There is some evidence to show that the presence of two or three islet autoantibodies predicts a faster deterioration of beta cell function (within 5 years).[28] If LADA is suspected, screening with GAD and ICA should be pursued. While the optimal treatment regimen has not been studied for the period between diagnosis and insulin dependency, many experts believe that insulin is the treatment of choice and should not be delayed. Our approach is to start with low-dose basal insulin and add mealtime rapid-acting insulin as postprandial readings indicate the need (see Chapter 2, p. 17).

Data suggest that insulin therapy can help to preserve C-peptide levels, although it does not seem to prevent the overall dependency on insulin earlier than those who are antibody-negative.[29] Use of other treatment agents is less clear, though evidence points to the avoidance of sulfonylurea use. One study showed that insulin-treated LADA patients had more persistent C-peptide levels compared to those treated with sulfonylureas.[30] Metformin use in LADA patients may not alter the outcome of insulin dependence,[24,25] and many LADA patients are started on metformin upon diagnosis of diabetes (as they are mistakenly classified as having type 2 diabetes). It may help to reduce glucose levels, but it also carries the risk of lactic acidosis in patients who are becoming insulin-deficient and ketosis-prone. Future therapies for LADA may be directed at prevention, specifically immunomodulation to halt beta-cell destruction (see Chapter 5, p. 53).

Recognition/Features in Adults with New-Onset Type 1/LADA

While all types of diabetes are diagnosed by blood glucose level, attention must be given to clues that indicate the presence of type 1 diabetes, as opposed to type 2, in an adult (Table 1.2). Commonly, adults are misclassified as having type 2 diabetes simply based upon their age. While type 2 diabetes

Table 1.2 Distinguishing Type 2 Diabetes from Type 1 Diabetes and LADA in Adults

	Type 2 More Likely	Type 1 More Likely	LADA More Likely
Physical examination findings	Central obesity with BMI >25 Acanthosis nigricans	Typically normal body weight (normal BMI)	Typically normal body weight (normal BMI)
Onset	Typically indolent	Typically abrupt Ketosis/DKA	Typically indolent
Family history	Common to have positive family history of type 2 diabetes	Occasionally positive family history of type 1 diabetes	Usually no family history
Autoantibodies	Negative GAD 65 autoantibodies	Positive GAD 65 autoantibodies	Positive GAD 65 autoantibodies
Other	Features of metabolic syndrome (high triglycerides, low HDL, and hypertension)	Presence of other autoimmune conditions (autoimmune thyroid disease, vitiligo, celiac disease, Addison's disease, autoimmune hepatitis, pernicious anemia)	Presence of other autoimmune conditions (autoimmune thyroid disease, vitiligo, celiac disease, Addison's disease, autoimmune hepatitis, pernicious anemia)

BMI, body mass index; DKA, diabetic ketoacidosis; GAD 65, glutamic acid decarboxylase 65.

is far more prevalent, recognition of type 1 is crucial to recognize, as treatment must be insulin.

Central obesity and acanthosis nigricans are physical examination findings usually indicating insulin resistance and type 2 diabetes. A family history of type 2 diabetes and findings such as low HDL cholesterol, elevated triglycerides, increased waist circumference, and hypertension indicate metabolic syndrome and a higher likelihood of type 2. An acute onset of hyperglycemia and ketosis should be recognized as features of type 1 diabetes in adults, although there are exceptions. There are ketosis-prone type 2 diabetics (often termed "Flatbush diabetes") who may present with diabetic ketoacidosis and an acute need for insulin, but who subsequently progress to a disease course of type 2 diabetes.[31] However, these patients typically do have features of insulin resistance.

In adults of normal body weight who lack features of insulin resistance and are treated with typical oral antidiabetic agents without improvement in their blood glucose readings, the clinician should suspect LADA. The prevalence of other autoimmune diseases should also arouse the suspicion of type 1 or LADA. Detection of autoantibodies can assist with diagnosis, and measuring ICAs and GAD is useful in distinguishing adult-onset type 1 diabetes and LADA from type 2 diabetes.[32]

References

1. American Diabetes Association. Diagnosis and Classification of Diabetes Mellitus. *Diabetes Care.* 2009;32:S62–S67.

2. International Expert Committee, ADA Workgroup Report. International Expert Committee Report on the Role of the A1C Assay in the Diagnosis of Diabetes. *Diabetes Care.* 2009;32(7):1327–1324.

3. Eisenbarth GS. Update in Type 1 diabetes. *J Clin Endocrinol Metab.* 2007;92(7):2403–2407.

4. Redondo MJ, Rewers M, Yu L, et al. Genetic determination of islet cell autoimmunity in monozygotic twin, dizygotic twin, and non-twin siblings of patients with type 1 diabetes; prospective twin study. *BMJ.* 1999;318:698–702.

5. Concannon P, Rich SS, Nepom GT. Genetics of type 1A diabetes. *N Engl J Med.* 2009;360(16):1646–1654.

6. Baisch JM, Weeks T, Giles R, et al. Analysis of HLA-DQ genotypes and susceptibility in insulin-dependent diabetes mellitus. *N Engl J Med.* 1990; 322(26):1836–1841.

7. Pugliese A. Genetics of type 1 diabetes. *Endocrinol Metab Clin North Am.* 2004;33:1–16.

8. Kavoura FK, Ioannidis JP. CTLA4 gene polymorphisms and susceptibility to type 1 diabetes mellitus: a HuGE review and meta-analysis. *Am J Epidemiol.* 2005;162(1):3–16.

9. Bach JF. The effect of infections on susceptibility to autoimmune and allergic diseases. *N Engl J Med.* 2002;347:911–920.

10. Couper JJ, Steele C, Beresford S, et al. Lack of association between duration of breast feeding or introduction of cow's milk and development of islet autoimmunity. *Diabetes.* 1999;48(11):2145–2149.

11. Hypponen E, Laara E, Reunanen A, et al. Intake of vitamin D and risk of type 1 diabetes: a birth cohort study. *Lancet.* 2001;358:1500–1503.

12. Ellis TM, Schatz DA, Ottendorfer EW, et al. The relationship between humoral and cellular immunity to IA-2 in IDDM. *Diabetes.* 1998;47(4):566–569.

13. Wang J, Miao D, Babu S, et al. Autoantibody-negative diabetes is not rare at all ages and increases with older age and obesity. *J Clin Endocrinol Metab.* 2007;92:88–92.

14. Barker JM. Clinical review: type 1 diabetes-associated autoimmunity: natural history, genetic associations, and screening. *J Clin Endocrinol Metab.* 2006;91(4):1210–1217.

15. Neufeld M, Maclaren NK, Blizzard RM. Two types of autoimmune Addison's disease associated with different polyglandular autoimmune (PGA) syndromes. *Medicine.* 1981;60:1653–1660.

16. Tisch R, McDevitt H. Insulin-dependent diabetes mellitus. *Cell.* 1996;85: 291–297.

17. Barker JM, Barriga KJ, Yu L. Prediction of autoantibody positivity and progression to type 1 diabetes: Diabetes Autoimmunity Study in the Young (DAISY). *J Clin Endocrinol Metab.* 2004;89(8):3896–3902.

18. Achenbach P, Bonifacio E, Koczwara K, Ziegler AG. Natural history of type 1 diabetes. *Diabetes.* 2005;54(Suppl 2):S25–S31.

19. Achenbach P, Warncke K, Reiter J, et al. Stratification of type 1 diabetes risk on the basis of islet autoantibody characteristics. *Diabetes.* 2004;53(2):384–392.

20. Barker JM, McFann K, Harrison LC, et al. Pre-type 1 diabetes dysmetabolism: maximal sensitivity achieved with both oral and intravenous glucose tolerance testing. *J Pediatr.* 2007;150:31–36.

21. Skyler JS. Update on worldwide efforts to prevent type 1 diabetes. *Ann NY Acad Sci.* 2008;1150:190–196.

22. Bingley PJ, Bonifacio E, Williams AJK, et al. Prediction of IDDM in the general population: strategies based on combination of autoantibody markers. *Diabetes.* 1997;46(11):1701–1710.

23. Turner R, Stratton I, Horton V, et al. UK Prospective Diabetes Study (UKPDS) Group: UKPDS 25: Autoantibodies to islet cell cytoplasm and glutamic acid decarboxylase for prediction of insulin requirement in type 2 diabetes. *Lancet.* 1997;350:1288–1293.

24. Leslie RDG, Williams R, Pozzilli P. Type 1 diabetes and latent autoimmune diabetes in adults: one end of the rainbow. *J Clin Endocrinol Metab.* 2006;91(5):1654–1659.

25. Pozzilli P, Di Marino U. Autoimmune diabetes not requiring insulin at diagnosis: latent autoimmune diabetes of the adult. *Diabetes Care.* 2001;24(8):1460–1467.

26. Palmer JP, Hampe CS, Chiu H, Goel A, Brooks-Worrell BM. Is latent autoimmune diabetes in adults distinct from type 1 diabetes or just type 1 diabetes at an older age? *Diabetes.* 2005;54(Suppl 2):S62–S67.

27. Diabetes Prevention Trial, Type 1 Diabetes Study Group. Effects of insulin in relatives of patients with type 1 diabetes mellitus. *N Engl J Med.* 2002;346(22):1685–691.

28. Stenstrom G, Gottsater A, Bakhtadze E, et al. Latent autoimmune diabetes in adults: definition, prevalence, β-cell function, and treatment. *Diabetes.* 2005;54(Suppl 2):S68–S72.

29. Davis TM, Wright AD, Mehta ZM, et al. Islet autoantibodies in clinically diagnosed type 2 diabetes; prevalence, and relationship with metabolic control (UKPDS 70). *Diabetologia.* 2005;48:695–702.

30. Moruyama T, Shimada A, Kanatsuka A, et al. Multicenter prevention trials of slowly progressive type 1 diabetes with small doses of insulin (the Kyoto Study). *Ann NY Acad Sci.* 2003;1005:362–369.

31. Umpierrez GE, Smiley D, Kitabchi AE. Narrative review: ketosis-prone type 2 diabetes mellitus. *Ann Intern Med.* 2006;144(5):350–357.

32. Littorn B, Sundkvist G, Hagopian W, et al. Islet cell and glutamic acid decarboxylase antibodies present at diagnosis of diabetes predict the need for insulin treatment. A cohort study in young adults whose disease was initially labeled as type 2 or unclassifiable diabetes. *Diabetes Care.* 1999;22:409–412.

Chapter 2

Management

Monitoring

Achieving normoglycemia safely requires the ability to monitor the results of insulin therapy. Patient self-monitoring of blood glucose (SMBG) provides immediate feedback on the current glucose level, whereas tests such as hemoglobin A1c provide information about the degree of control over a longer period.

SMBG

SMBG is recommended at least three times a day, although many patients need to test more often to achieve adequate control.[1] Patients should test more often during illness, exercise, or other conditions that may cause hyper- or hypoglycemia. Numerous blood glucose meters are available commercially. Some meters require chip insertion or entry of a code corresponding to the batch of test strips in use; if the correct code is not entered, the results may be less accurate. Meters should be calibrated periodically using control solutions.

Many glucose meters are designed to work with capillary blood from sites other than the fingertip (e.g., forearm) which may be less painful. However, testing should be done using the fingertip at times of rapid blood glucose level change (e.g., after meals) or when hypoglycemia is suspected, since alternative sites may provide less accurate results in such situations.[2,3]

Generally, patients being treated with intensive insulin therapy need to test before and 2 hours after meals to provide enough results for appropriate adjustment of their insulin regimens. SMBG results can be analyzed more easily when they are recorded in columns corresponding to before and after each meal, thereby enabling recognition of trends or patterns for specific meals or times of day. The results from many meters can also be downloaded into a computer to provide similar visualization of trends and variability.

A1c

The most widely used measure of chronic glycemic control is the A1c, known variably as glycated hemoglobin, glycohemoglobin, hemoglobin A1c, or HbA1c, depending in part on the assay used. Red blood cells are freely permeable to glucose, and as hemoglobin is exposed to glucose it becomes irreversibly bound to glucose in a glucose-concentration-dependent manner. The percentage of hemoglobin thus bound to glucose correlates to the average blood glucose concentration during the lifetime of the red cells and is reported as the A1c.

Although the average lifespan of red cells is 120 days, the A1c best reflects blood glucose levels over the previous 2 to 3 months.

Various factors that affect hemoglobin or red cell survival can likewise affect A1c results, rendering them less accurate as measures of glycemic control. High erythrocyte turnover, as in acute blood loss, hemolytic anemia, or treatment with erythropoietin, results in misleadingly low A1c results, whereas processes that prolong erythrocyte survival, such as iron deficiency anemia, result in misleadingly high A1c results. Intake of large amounts of vitamin C or vitamin E can falsely lower or elevate results. Some A1c assays are also affected by hemoglobin variants such as HbS (sickle cell trait).[4] Transfusions and chronic kidney or liver disease may also affect A1c results.

Estimated Average Glucose (eAG)

An international study recently examined the relationship between A1c values and mean blood glucose and found that a simple linear relationship exists between them over a clinically relevant glycemic range.[5] The A1c can be converted to an estimated average glucose (eAG) using the formula $eAG_{mg/dL}$ = 28.7 × A1c − 46.7 or $eAG_{mmol/L}$ = 1.59 × A1c − 2.59. Table 2.1 shows sample equivalent values.

The vast majority of A1c assays worldwide have been standardized, but a new, more stable and specific measurement method has been developed and proposed for global standardization.[6,7] The new method produces numerical results 1.5 to 2.0 percentage points lower than the current method, and the results are reported in millimoles per mole of total hemoglobin rather than a percentage. To avoid confusion, it is proposed that in the future results will be reported with three values: the familiar A1c value, an eAG derived from that result, and the result according to the new method in mmol/mol.[8]

Table 2.1 A1c and Corresponding eAG Values

A1c (%)	eAG	
	mg/dL	mmol/L
5.0	97	5.4
6.0	126	7.0
6.5	140	7.8
7.0	154	8.6
7.5	169	9.4
8.0	183	10.2
8.5	197	11.0
9.0	212	11.8
9.5	226	12.6
10.0	240	13.4
11.0	269	14.9
12.0	298	16.5

Fructosamine

Fructosamine refers to a group of glycated serum proteins, predominantly albumin, that form in a similar way to glycated hemoglobin. However, because serum albumin has a shorter half-life than hemoglobin, the serum fructosamine level reflects the degree of glycemic control over the preceding 2 to 3 weeks.[9,10] Measurement of fructosamine may be useful when an estimate of very recent glycemic control is desired or when the A1c may be inaccurate or is discordant with the patient's SMBG results.

Fructosamine generally correlates to A1c, although within-subject variation is greater.[11–13] Furthermore, as with A1c, various physiologic effects interfere with its reliability as an indicator of glycemic control; the fructosamine measurement will be misleadingly low if the serum albumin concentration is low or if there is rapid albumin turnover, as with hepatic disease, protein-losing enteropathy, or the nephrotic syndrome.[14]

Ketones

Patients should test their urine for ketones using commercially available ketone strips during acute illness or stress, when blood glucose levels are consistently elevated (>300 mg/dL [>16.7 mmol/L]), or with any symptoms of diabetic ketoacidosis (DKA) (e.g., nausea, vomiting, abdominal pain).[1] Ketonuria may not indicate impending DKA. Positive results can occur during fasting or periods of negative caloric balance and in pregnancy. Other situations warrant repeat testing every few hours, extra insulin, and fluid intake to ensure adequate hydration. If the ketonuria does not resolve or if there is a suspicion of ketoacidosis, the patient should seek evaluation at an emergency department.

Continuous Glucose Monitoring

SMBG with fingerstick testing is a vital part of successful management of type 1 diabetes, but it is inconvenient and uncomfortable and provides the glucose level only at the time of testing. Despite testing several times a day, patients may have periods of asymptomatic hypo- or hyperglycemia. Continuous glucose monitoring (CGM) offers patients the ability to monitor their blood glucose continuously with minimal effort. The currently available systems use a device that adheres to the skin and includes a small catheter inserted with an introducer needle. Once inserted, the needle is removed and the catheter remains in the subcutaneous tissue, allowing the device to sample the interstitial fluid. The device also includes a transmitter that sends a glucose measurement every minute or 5 minutes (depending on the system) to a receiver, which displays the result along with a graph of recent results and an indicator showing the direction and rate of change. A new device is inserted every 3 to 7 days.

Currently available sensors allow glycemic thresholds to be set; a glucose level beyond these thresholds triggers an alarm to alert the patient of hypo- or hyperglycemia so that action can be taken before the condition worsens. Thus, they are useful for preventing overnight hypoglycemia and unexpected daytime hypo- or hyperglycemia, and may be particularly useful for patients with hypoglycemic unawareness (see Chapter 3) or those whose fear of hypoglycemia limits the achievement of tight glycemic control.

CGM is also available for short-term diagnostic use in a form that stores glucose data for later download without displaying the information to the patient. Such a device could be used in a patient with a high A1c despite seemingly good SMBG results to detect periods of hyperglycemia occurring at times when the patient is not performing SMBG.

CGM does not eliminate the need for fingerstick glucose monitoring. The sensors must be calibrated at least daily to a fingerstick result. Sensors are not as accurate as fingerstick testing, and therefore fingerstick testing is still recommended before making management decisions.[15] Furthermore, since the sensors measure the interstitial fluid glucose concentration rather than the blood glucose level, during periods of rapid change in glucose level the sensor readings may lag behind the blood glucose level.[16]

There is growing recognition that the amount of glycemic variability, like the average glucose (indicated by the A1c), may have consequences.[17] There is evidence of endothelial damage, but the extent to which glycemic variability leads to micro- and macrovascular complications remains controversial.[18–20] Studies have shown benefits from CGM in both variability and A1c. In a recent trial, patients 25 years of age or older using CGM had A1c values 0.53 lower on average than matched patients performing SMBG alone (average 6.6 times per day) after 26 weeks without an increase in hypoglycemic events and had a significantly greater amount of time per day within the target glucose range of 71 to 180 mg/dL.[21] Other studies have demonstrated a decreased incidence of hypoglycemic and hyperglycemic episodes with CGM, although without an additional reduction in A1c.[22,23] CGM systems are expensive, but as their benefits become more established, coverage by insurance companies is increasing.

Diabetes Education and Nutrition

Diabetes self-management education (DSME) is necessary for all patients with type 1 diabetes and can improve patient outcomes.[24] All patients should be referred to qualified educators at the time of diagnosis and periodically for continued management skills or with changes in their treatment plan to update their knowledge and skills in coping with and managing their diabetes.

Diabetes educators are those with education in diabetes management and counseling. Certified Diabetes Educators (CDEs) are educators who are certified by the National Certification Board for Diabetes Educators (NCBDE), have demonstrated core knowledge and experience, and have passed a certifying examination. Educators can provide basic training, such as defining glucose goals and teaching recognition and treatment of hypoglycemia, to more complex care, such as adjusting insulin for exercise and assisting in insulin pump training.

The American Diabetes Association publishes standards of care for diabetes education[25] to define quality diabetes self-management education and to help educators provide evidence-based education and care, and the American

Association of Diabetes Educators provides a list of CDEs by locations (see Chapter 6).

Medical nutrition therapy (MNT) is an integral part of diabetes education. In patients with type 1 diabetes, MNT provided by a registered dietitian can result in a 1% reduction in A1c.[26]

As reviewed in the next section, insulin therapy should approximate normal physiologic insulin secretion. Mealtime insulin should be dosed based on the carbohydrate content of meals and snacks. Patients need nutrition education to understand the carbohydrate content of meals, to learn how to dose their insulin for meal content, and to ensure adequate nutritional intake. We recommend the use of an insulin-to-carbohydrate-gram ratio, but some patients use a carbohydrate exchange system, which also may work well. If individuals are on fixed insulin doses (either premixed insulin or a set amount of rapid-acting insulin before each meal), then their carbohydrate intake should be kept consistent to prevent hypo- and hyperglycemia.

Nutrition recommendations for the general population are advised for those with type 1 diabetes, including limiting saturated fat to less than 7% of total calories, minimizing trans fat intake, protein intake of 15% to 20% for those with normal renal function, and consuming a variety of fiber-containing foods.[27] There does not seem to be a benefit from vitamin or mineral supplementation in those without deficiencies,[27] with the exception of certain populations and circumstances (such as folate use in pregnancy and calcium to prevent osteoporosis).

Insulin Therapy

Insulin therapy forms the core of type 1 diabetes management, but many additional elements are a part of the comprehensive care needed for a successful outcome. These elements include[24]:

- Comprehensive history and physical examination
- Evaluation of eating patterns, weight, nutrition knowledge, exercise habits
- Evaluation of glycemic control, including A1c and SMBG as discussed above
- Screening for complications, including hypoglycemia, hypoglycemic unawareness, and diabetic ketoacidosis (see Chapter 3)
- Laboratory tests: see Table 2.2 and Chapter 3 for details
- Referrals for annual dilated eye examination, registered dietitian for MNT, diabetes self-management education, dental examination, and mental health professional, if needed

See Table 2.2 for a summary of American Diabetes Association recommendations.

Intensive Insulin Therapy

Since the Diabetes Control and Complications Trial[28] demonstrated considerable reductions in complications with intensive insulin therapy, intensive insulin

Table 2.2 Summary of American Diabetes Association Recommendations[24]

Glycemic goals	
A1c	Goal <7.0% *in general.* Measure semiannually if at goal with stable therapy, quarterly if not at goal or therapy has changed.
Preprandial glucose	70–130 mg/dL (3.9–7.2 mmol/L)
Peak postprandial glucose	<180 mg/dL (<10.0 mmol/L)
Blood pressure	<130/80 mm Hg
Fasting lipid profile	At least annually
LDL cholesterol	<100 mg/dL (<70 mg/dL optional)
HDL cholesterol	>40 mg/dL in men, >50 mg/dL in women
Triglycerides	<150 mg/dL
Serum creatinine	At least annually with estimated glomerular filtration rate
Albumin:creatinine ratio	Annually; if positive, repeat twice within 3–6 months
Thyroid-stimulating hormone	Every 1–2 years
Celiac disease screening: tissue transglutaminase or antiendomysial antibodies	At diagnosis and again if gastrointestinal symptoms develop
Dilated eye examination	Annually
Comprehensive foot examination	Annually

therapy has become the standard therapy for type 1 diabetes. Intensive insulin therapy seeks to replicate normal insulin physiology as closely as possible with multiple daily injections of insulin. There are three components to this therapy[29]:

• Basal insulin: mimics the constant release of insulin that regulates lipolysis and hepatic glucose output

• Prandial or bolus insulin: mimics the usual response of endogenous insulin to food intake

• Correction-dose or supplemental insulin: addresses pre-meal or between-meal hyperglycemia independently of the prandial insulin

A combination of insulin types is used to construct a regimen with these components. The onset, peak, and duration of action of commonly used insulins are shown in Table 2.3, and their idealized time-action profiles are depicted in Figure 2.1. These are general values and vary between and within patients depending on dose injected, site of administration, skin temperature, and other variables.

Basal Insulin

The prolonged peakless activity of insulin glargine (Lantus) makes it ideal for use as basal insulin. It is generally given once daily at bedtime or in the morning;

Table 2.3 Duration of Action of Frequently Used Insulins and Insulin Analogs[29]

Type	Name	Onset	Peak	Duration
Rapid-acting	Lispro, aspart, glulisine	5–15 min	30–90 min	4–6 h
Short-acting	Regular	30–60 min	2–3 h	6–10 h
Intermediate-acting	NPH	2–4 h	4–10 h	12–18 h
Long-acting	Detemir	2–4 h	3–14 h*	6–23 h
Long-acting	Glargine	2–4 h	None	20–24 h

*The peak serum concentration occurs at 6–8 h, but the peak in effect is slight, with >50% of its maximum effect occurring at 3–14 h.

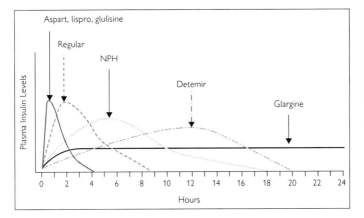

Figure 2.1. Idealized time-action profiles of frequently used insulins and insulin analogs. Republished with permission from "Management of Type 1 Diabetes," by IB Hirsh and JS Skyler, in www.endotext.org, version 21 September 2009.

it should be given at the same time each day. In some patients its action wanes earlier than in most, necessitating twice-daily dosing. Insulin detemir (Levemir) is another option for basal insulin. It is classified as a long-acting insulin, although at low doses its duration of action more closely resembles NPH, and for patients with type 1 diabetes it should be given twice daily to ensure adequate 24-hour activity. NPH insulin given twice daily can also be used as basal insulin.

Insulin glargine appears to result in fewer episodes of nocturnal hypoglycemia compared to NPH, which may allow further titration of dose to yield lower fasting glucose levels, although a decrease in A1c from glargine versus NPH has not been consistently demonstrated.[29,30] Insulin detemir has also been shown to produce less nocturnal hypoglycemia and also less weight gain than NPH.[31]

Prandial Insulin

The rapid onset and short duration of action of the rapid-acting insulin analogs make them well suited for use as prandial insulin. Three rapid-acting insulin analogs are currently available: aspart (Novolog), lispro (Humalog), and glulisine (Apidra). Regular insulin has also been used as the prandial insulin, but it has several disadvantages compared with the rapid-acting analogs. The rapid-acting analogs have been shown to reduce postprandial hyperglycemia more than regular insulin and to cause hypoglycemia less often than regular insulin. These effects reduce glycemic variability, although reductions in A1c compared to regular have generally been modest.[29,32–35] Furthermore, the recommended timing of regular insulin administration is less convenient; for optimal control of the prandial blood glucose spike, regular insulin should be taken 30 minutes before the meal, requiring advance planning, whereas rapid-acting analogs are taken immediately before eating.

Correction-Dose Insulin

The rapid-acting analogs are also well suited for use as supplemental insulin to correct hyperglycemia. They lower blood glucose more rapidly than regular insulin and do not have as prolonged an effect.[36]

Older Insulin Regimens

Older conventional insulin regimens typically consisted of an injection of regular insulin combined with NPH insulin before breakfast and another combined dose before dinner; sometimes this second dose was split, with the regular given before dinner and the NPH before bed to reduce the risk of nighttime hypoglycemia. Due to the peak of NPH and the extended duration of regular, both insulins provide basal and prandial effects, complicating adjustments to the regimen and necessitating strict consistency of the timing of injections and meals. Using a rapid-acting analog as the prandial insulin allows patients to skip meals or change mealtimes without risking hypo- or hyperglycemia. Although more injections are required with intensive insulin therapy than conventional therapy, most patients with type 1 diabetes prefer the dietary freedom.[37] Furthermore, the use of insulin pens rather than vials and syringes makes taking injections quick and easy while on the go.

Constructing a Regimen

Initial insulin doses are often based on a patient's total daily dose, which typically ranges from 0.3 to 0.7 units/kg. A total daily dose can be estimated from a patient's current insulin regimen or from a patient's weight, using 0.3 to 0.5 units/kg to start. Half of this total is typically given as basal insulin, either as a single dose of glargine or divided as two doses of detemir or NPH. The other half of the total daily dose is given as prandial insulin, divided between the meals eaten.

Rather than taking the same amount of insulin with each meal, patients should adjust their prandial doses according to the amount of carbohydrate to be consumed. Ideally, patients should learn to count carbohydrates (i.e., learn to estimate the amount of carbohydrates in grams of their meal) and use that estimate with an insulin-to-carbohydrate ratio to calculate a dose of prandial insulin tailored to their meal. An insulin-to-carbohydrate ratio can be estimated by dividing 500 by the total daily insulin requirement. For example, a patient taking a total of 42 units a day would have an insulin-to-carbohydrate ratio of about 1:12. That patient would take 1 unit of insulin for every 12 g carbohydrate consumed, and so to calculate a prandial insulin dose the patient would divide the amount of carbohydrate to be eaten by 12.

The supplemental dose can be estimated by dividing 1,700 by the total daily insulin requirement. The result is an estimate of the patient's sensitivity to insulin (i.e., the expected decrease in blood glucose [in mg/dL] from 1 unit of insulin).[38] For example, if a patient uses an average of 32 units daily, the sensitivity or correction factor is 53. To use this figure, the patient would subtract a goal glucose (e.g., 100 mg/dL) from the current blood glucose and divide the difference by the correction factor, yielding the needed supplemental dose to correct the hyperglycemia. For example, if the same patient's blood glucose is 260 mg/dL: 260 − 100 = 160; 160 ÷ 53 = 3 supplemental units needed. The supplemental dose can be calculated before each meal when the patient has hyperglycemia and can be added to the prandial dose. If the patient is not eating at the time the blood glucose is tested, the patient would take the supplemental dose alone.

When using insulin in this manner, it is important to consider how much insulin is still active from previous doses. Adding additional doses before previous doses have had their full effect ("insulin stacking") can cause hypoglycemia. As a rough guideline, a supplemental dose given less than 3 hours after another dose can be halved to avoid this effect.[37]

Various methods of estimating insulin-to-carbohydrate ratios and correction factors have been devised and compared.[39] Regardless of how the initial regimen is devised, it should be reassessed and adjusted until appropriate glycemic control is achieved. The basal insulin dose is best adjusted based on fasting blood glucose levels and the prandial and supplemental doses based on evaluation of blood glucose readings before and 2 hours after the doses were given. Insulin-to-carbohydrate ratios can be adjusted similarly according to blood glucose readings before and after meals in which the exact number of carbohydrates was known. Interpreting blood glucose records and adjusting the regimen appropriately often becomes complicated. Many factors can cause variability in glycemic control, including insulin absorption rate (affected by skin temperature, exercise, and injection site), food absorption rate (affected by nutrient content, autonomic dysfunction, and medications), exercise, stress, and hormonal changes (such as menstrual cycles).[40]

Glycemic Goals

The American Diabetes Association recommends an A1c goal for nonpregnant adults in general of less than 7%. This goal should be individualized. Clinical trials have demonstrated a small but incremental benefit in microvascular disease prevention from lowering A1c from 7% to 6%. However, doing so substantially elevates the risk of hypoglycemia, and thus in setting a target for an individual patient the benefits of microvascular disease prevention must be weighed against the added risk of hypoglycemia. The lower goal is especially appropriate, if it can be met without inducing significant hypoglycemia, for patients with a short duration of diabetes, long life expectancy, and little comorbidity, as such patients are more likely to benefit from the reduced complication risk. Conversely, a higher A1c goal may be appropriate for patients with a history of severe hypoglycemia or hypoglycemic unawareness, limited life expectancy, or extensive comorbidities.[24]

In addition to A1c goals, the American Diabetes Association recommends preprandial and peak postprandial targets (see Table 2.2). The A1c is the primary target; the other targets correlate to the achievement of an A1c below 7%. Both preprandial and postprandial glucose levels contribute to the A1c, with a higher relative contribution from the latter at A1c levels close to 7%. Thus, both components should be considered when assessing glycemic control.[24]

Practical Considerations

Vials or pens of insulin not in use should be stored in a refrigerator. Insulin in use can be kept at room temperature, but extreme temperatures (<36° or >86°F [<2° or >30°C]) and excessive agitation should be avoided. Insulin potency may decline after a vial or pen has been in use for more than 1 month, particularly if it was stored at room temperature. The insulin should be inspected for color or clarity changes, clumping, or precipitation before each use.

If concurrent administration of rapid- or short-acting and NPH insulin is desired, the two insulins can be mixed in the same syringe (the NPH should be added second), but insulin glargine should not be mixed with other insulins. Air bubbles in an insulin syringe or pen may increase injection discomfort and may cause underdelivery of insulin from a pen. Patients using premixed insulins such as Novolin 70/30 or Humulin 50/50 should gently roll the vial between their hands before filling the syringe to ensure adequate mixing of the components.

Insulin may be injected into the subcutaneous tissue of the upper arm and the anterior and lateral aspects of the thigh, buttocks, and abdomen, except within 5 cm of the navel. Absorption is fastest in the abdomen; thus, if multiple sites are used, the rapid- or short-acting insulin is best injected into the abdomen and the intermediate- or long-acting insulin into the other site. Rotation of injection location is important to prevent lipohypertrophy or lipoatrophy, but to minimize variability due to differing absorption rates, rotation should occur within a site rather than between sites.[40]

Continuous Subcutaneous Insulin Infusion (CSII; Insulin Pumps)

Continuous subcutaneous insulin infusion (CSII) using an insulin pump is an alternative to multiple daily injections. The same principles of intensive insulin therapy and physiologic insulin replacement apply to CSII, except that, rather than using separate insulins for the basal and prandial/correction components of therapy, a single insulin continuously infused at varying rates provides all components of therapy. The pump infuses insulin continuously at a low rate, typically 0.2 to 1 unit per hour, for basal insulin. Superimposed on the basal insulin are manually activated boluses at mealtime or as supplemental insulin for hyperglycemia.

Most pump systems include a pump unit, which comprises an insulin reservoir with pump mechanism, battery, and control panel. The reservoir is attached to a long flexible catheter or tubing that leads to an infusion device. The infusion device is a relatively flat piece of plastic that includes a small plastic catheter through which insulin is infused after being inserted into the subcutaneous tissue at any location appropriate for insulin injections. This device remains in place for 2 to 3 days, after which the location must be changed to ensure adequate insulin infusion.

The rapid-acting analogs are the preferred insulins for use in pumps. They have been shown to reduce A1c slightly more than regular insulin when used in pumps.[41] Some studies have also shown a lower rate of hypoglycemia with the analogs.[29,42,43]

Patients typically require about 20% less insulin per day when the insulin is delivered by pump rather than multiple injections.[44] Thus, when switching a patient from multiple injections to a pump, the insulin doses must be reduced accordingly. Typically about half of the adjusted total daily insulin dose is given as basal insulin and the other half split among the meals. The basal rates, carbohydrate ratios, and sensitivity factor are adjusted empirically according to the patient's blood glucose monitoring results.

CSII offers a variety of benefits. Pumps offer more flexibility than multiple injection regimens. The basal insulin infusion rate can be customized and programmed to vary throughout the day, unlike insulin glargine, which provides relatively constant insulin activity. A pump could be set to deliver a higher basal rate in the morning and a lower basal rate overnight, and it could also be set to increase or decrease the basal rate temporarily by a certain proportion. For example, during exercise a pump could be set to deliver 50% of the usual basal rate to prevent hypoglycemia.

Pumps also offer more convenience. A bolus of insulin is activated by pressing a few buttons rather than preparing an insulin syringe or pen; no injection is needed. Furthermore, the pump does the calculations to determine the appropriate bolus dose once the patient's insulin-to-carbohydrate ratio and correction factor are programmed. The patient need only enter the current blood glucose and the amount of carbohydrate to be consumed; the pump will calculate the appropriate prandial insulin and supplemental correction insulin doses.

Pumps may offer improved glycemic control. One meta-analysis showed that CSII (using a variety of insulins) resulted in a 0.53% reduction in A1c and less glycemic variability compared with multiple injections.[45] Subsequent studies comparing CSII with multiple daily injections using insulin analogs have also shown lower A1c[46] and lower fructosamine without an increased risk of hypoglycemia.[47] A recent meta-analysis concluded that CSII modestly reduced A1c without significant differences in hypoglycemia compared to multiple injections.[48] However, a recent trial comparing the two treatment modalities in type 1 diabetes patients naïve to intensive insulin therapy showed no difference in glycemic control.[49]

In terms of safety, pump therapy has some advantages and disadvantages. Current pumps have programs that allow the pump to calculate the active "insulin on board" to avoid insulin stacking if a bolus is requested within a few hours of a previous bolus. The pump thus subtracts the active insulin from the calculated correction and/or prandial dose and delivers just the difference rather than the full dose, which would likely cause hypoglycemia if not adjusted. This feature likely contributes to the lower rates of hypoglycemia sometimes seen with CSII. Pump therapy also entails some specific risks; undetected interruptions in insulin infusion, whether due to kinked tubing or pump failure, may lead to ketotic episodes more often and more quickly than with injection therapy, and infections or inflammation at the infusion site may occur.[50]

Patients sometimes have misconceptions about insulin pumps, thinking that pumps "do everything" for them. In fact, while pumps provide great flexibility, they require patients to devote considerable attention to their diabetes. Patients must always test their blood glucose at least several times a day. For optimal results, the patient should be adept at carbohydrate counting and have a clear understanding of the components of intensive insulin therapy. Candidates for CSII must be strongly motivated to improve glucose control and be willing to assume substantial responsibility for their day-to-day care. The necessary attention may be too demanding for some individuals. CSII therapy should be prescribed, implemented, and followed by a skilled professional team familiar with CSII therapy and capable of supporting the patient.[50]

Amylin and Pramlintide

Amylin is a beta-cell hormone that is co-located and co-secreted with insulin, playing a complementary role by regulating the rate of glucose secretion during the postprandial period. It does so through several mechanisms of action: slowing gastric emptying, suppressing inappropriate postprandial glucagon secretion, and regulating food intake.[51] Patients with type 1 diabetes have insulin and amylin deficiency; therefore, besides giving these patients insulin, adding amylin could potentially benefit many of them through its mechanisms of action. Amylin has not been pursued as a pharmacologic preparation due to its low solubility and a propensity to aggregate. Pramlintide (Symlin) is a synthetic, soluble, nonaggregating analog of amylin with similar mechanisms of action that collectively regulate the glucose levels in the circulation following meals.

Pramlintide is approved for use only in patients who are taking mealtime insulin. Pramlintide precipitates above a pH of 5.5 and must be injected separately from insulin at a different site.[52] The optimal timing for administration is immediately before a meal. Preprandial insulin dosages (including premixed insulin) should be reduced by 30% to 50% and should subsequently be titrated upward to achieve euglycemia once the target pramlintide dosage is reached.

Pramlintide is currently available in vials and pens. The recommended starting dosage for type 1 diabetes is 15 µg before each meal, with increases in 15-µg increments every 3 to 7 days, as tolerated, to a goal of 60 µg. Persistent nausea should prompt backward titration until it is resolved.

Mild to moderate nausea is the most commonly reported side effect and generally dissipates by the fourth week on pramlintide.[53] Nausea can be minimized by slow upward dose titration. Hypoglycemia can occur if mealtime insulin is not reduced appropriately when pramlintide is initiated; insulin-induced hypoglycemia typically occurs within 3 hours following pramlintide injection. Pramlintide should not be administered to patients with severe hypoglycemia unawareness. Pramlintide should be administered only before meals that contain at least 250 calories or 30 g of carbohydrates. Patients may need to administer prandial insulin after meals until they become familiar with the degree of satiety and resulting reduction of carbohydrate intake that may occur.

Pramlintide slows gastric emptying and may delay the rate of absorption of oral medications. Patients with gastroparesis should not use pramlintide. Oral medications that require rapid absorption for effectiveness should be administered either 1 hour before or 2 hours after the injection of pramlintide.

Special Situations

Sick Days

Acute illness typically results in hyperglycemia due to elevations in counterregulatory hormones. Occasionally, patients may also become hypoglycemic when ill. The best strategy is to have patients frequently monitor their blood glucose and ketones, drink adequate amounts of fluids, and ingest carbohydrates during illness. To prevent starvation ketosis, ingestion of 150 to 200 g carbohydrate daily (45 to 50 g every 3 to 4 hours) should be sufficient.[54]

Type 1 diabetic patients must receive education about the importance of basal insulin and the risk of DKA if insulin is held. Many patients, when ill or having decreased appetite, nausea, or vomiting, tend to hold all of their insulin for fear of hypoglycemia. This creates the potential for DKA or worsening hyperglycemia. Patients must continue to administer basal insulin. For the insulin pump patient, a temporary increased basal rate should be set for hyperglycemia associated with illness (an increase of 20% to 30%), with continued SMBG and supplemental or correction insulin as glucose levels warrant. For patients on injections, basal insulin must be continued, and higher doses of rapid-acting insulin may need to be given at 3- to 4-hour intervals.

Exercise

Although exercise has not been shown to improve glycemic control in type 1 diabetes, it can improve lipids and blood pressure and increase cardiovascular fitness. Patients with type 1 diabetes should exercise as part of a healthy lifestyle. However, patients should be assessed for their level of glucose control and presence of complications before starting an exercise program.[55]

With exercise, patients may experience hypo- or hyperglycemia. This can be problematic to exercise performance and can become a source of anxiety for patients. Multiple factors play into the metabolic response to exercise, including the duration, intensity, and type of exercise, as well as the glucose level, the amount and types of insulin on board, and the amount of food ingested before exercise.[56]

Some patients experience hyperglycemia with exercise as a result of catecholamine release and sympathetic nervous system activation. SMBG before, during, and after exercise is recommended to see what the individual effects are, and this information can be used to calculate insulin adjustments or the need for additional carbohydrate intake. Patients with blood glucose levels above 250 mg/dL or positive ketones should avoid exercise and should get prompt evaluation.

More common, and more feared by patients, is the experience of hypoglycemia. The hepatic counterregulatory response to hypoglycemia may not occur during exercise in patients on exogenous insulin (see Chapter 3, p. 37). Hypoglycemia can occur during exercise, or up to 12 to 24 hours after exercise is complete.[56] Carbohydrate-based foods should be readily available during and after physical activity. For planned exercise, a reduction in insulin and/or an increase in carbohydrate intake prior to exercise is recommended.

Patients on insulin pumps have more flexibility in changing their basal insulin. While this may not be needed for short periods of exercise, it may be necessary for longer periods of activity (>60 minutes). Basal rates can be lowered from 20% to 50%, but these changes should be made 1 to 3 hours prior to exercise to be effective due to active insulin time. For mild or moderate exercise over shorter periods, the bolus dose with the meal prior to exercise can be reduced by 30% to 50%. Patients on injections can also reduce their bolus dose with the meal prior to exercise (decrease by 30% to 50%) or reduce their long-acting insulin by 20% to 50%. Again, the best strategy seems one of trial and error: frequent SMBG to learn individual patterns and responses to exercise, then trying alterations in amounts of insulin or food intake to counteract any hypo- or hyperglycemic responses.[56]

For unplanned exercise, carbohydrates should be ingested before activity. More carbohydrates may be needed for more intense exercise, and again, more individualized plans can be determined with careful SMBG.[57]

Travel

Traveling can cause stress, anxiety, and fluctuations in glucose control. Meals can be delayed, food selections may be limited, and activity levels can be increased. Planning in advance can avoid much of the stress associated with traveling in insulin-treated patients. A good rule is to pack double the supplies that are anticipated for travel and to remember that insulin, test strips, and glucometers should be kept away from extremes of temperatures.

Patients should perform frequent SMBG and stay hydrated. In traveling across time zones, it is important to pay attention to the basal insulin dosing schedule so that basal doses are not missed, leading to periods of insulin deficiency. This can be done by keeping track of the home time zone and continuing to dose based on the usual home schedule, or splitting the basal insulin dose in half and taking it every 12 hours.[58] Insulin pump patients can set the new time zone time into their pumps.

Type 1 patients should familiarize themselves with the most recent recommendations and guidelines for air travel and airport security.[59] At security checkpoints, patients should notify the security officer that they are diabetic and have diabetes-related supplies. Medications and diabetes supplies should be in carry-on baggage, and all supplies needed to care for diabetes should be permitted once they go through screening. As an extra precaution, patients should bring their prescriptions for medications and supplies. Medications should be labeled, and insulin pumps and pump supplies must be accompanied by insulin. Insulin, glucometers, and insulin pumps are safe to go through x-ray devices.

Alcohol

The same precautions that apply to the general population regarding alcohol use apply to those with type 1 diabetes: adult men should have no more than two drinks per day, adult women no more than one per day.[27] All patients should be cautioned that alcohol use can increase the risk of hypoglycemia, as the metabolism of alcohol can impair gluconeogenesis, and alcohol use may mask the symptoms of hypoglycemia.[67] If patients with type 1 diabetes choose to drink alcohol, food should be consumed concurrently to help avoid hypoglycemia. Blood glucose should be monitored more frequently, and a bedtime snack is recommended. For CSII patients, basal rates can be lowered by 20%. Patients should also be aware that excessive use of alcohol or ingesting alcohol with carbohydrate mixers can cause hyperglycemia.

References

1. American Diabetes Association. Tests of glycemia in diabetes. *Diabetes Care.* 2004;27(Suppl 1):S91–93.

2. Ellison JM, Stegmann JM, Colner SL. Rapid changes in postprandial blood glucose produce concentration differences at finger, forearm, and thigh sampling sites. *Diabetes Care.* 2002;25:961–964.

3. Jungheim K, Koschinsky T. Glucose monitoring at the arm: risky delays of hypoglycemia and hyperglycemia detection. *Diabetes Care.* 2002;25:956–960.

4. National Diabetes Information Clearinghouse (NDIC). Sickle Cell Trait and Other Hemoglobinopathies and Diabetes: Important Information for Physicians. NIH Publication No. 09–6287, November 2008. Available at http://diabetes.niddk. nih.gov/dm/pubs/hemovari-A1C/SickleCell-Fact.pdf. Accessed 16 Sept 2009.

5. Nathan DM, Kuenen J, Borg R, et al. Translating the A1C assay into estimated average glucose values. *Diabetes Care.* 2008;31:1473–1478.

6. Jeppsson JO, Kobold U, Barr J, et al. Approved IFCC reference method for the measurement of HbA1c in human blood. *Clin Chem Lab Med.* 2002;40:78–89.

7. Sacks DB and the ADA/EASD/IDF Working Group of the HbA1c Assay. Global harmonization of hemoglobin A1c. *Clin Chem.* 2005;51:681–683.

8. Kahn R, Fonseca V. Translating the A1C assay. *Diabetes Care.* 2008;31:1704–1707.

9. Armbruster DA. Fructosamine: structure, analysis, and clinical usefulness. *Clin Chem.* 1987;33:2153–2163.

10. Takahashi S, Uchino H, Shimizu T, et al. Comparison of glycated albumin (GA) and glycated hemoglobin (HbA1c) in type 2 diabetic patients: usefulness of GA for evaluation of short-term changes in glycemic control. *Endocrinol J.* 2007;54:139–144.

11. Baker JR, Metcalf PA, Holdaway IM, Johnson RN. Serum fructosamine concentration as measure of blood glucose control in type I (insulin-dependent) diabetes mellitus. *Br Med J (Clin Res Ed).* 1985;290:352–355.

12. Narbonne H, Renacco E, Pradel V, Portugal H, Vialettes B. Can fructosamine be a surrogate for HbA1c in evaluating the achievement of therapeutic goals in diabetes? *Diabetes Metab.* 2001;27:598–603.

13. Howey JE, Bennet WM, Browning MC, Jung RT, Fraser CG. Clinical utility of assays of glycosylated haemoglobin and serum fructosamine compared: use of data on biological variation. *Diabet Med.* 1989;6:793–796.

14. Howey JE, Browning MC, Fraser CG. Assay of serum fructosamine that minimizes standardization and matrix problems: use to assess components of biological variation. *Clin Chem.* 1987;33(2 Pt 1):269–272.

15. Kovatchev B, Anderson S, Heinmann L, Clarke W. Comparison of the numerical and clinical accuracy of four continuous glucose monitors. *Diabetes Care.* 2008;31:1160–1164.

16. Monsod TP, Flanagan DE, Rife F, Saenz R. Do sensor glucose levels accurately predict plasma glucose concentrations during hypoglycemia and hyperinsulinemia? *Diabetes Care.* 2002;25:889–893.

17. Hirsch IB. Glycemic variability: it's not just about A1C anymore! *Diabetes Technol Ther.* 2005;7:780–783.

18. Monnier L, Mas E, Ginet C, et al. Activation of oxidative stress by acute glucose fluctuations compared with sustained chronic hyperglycemia in patients with type 2 diabetes. *JAMA.* 2006;295:1681–1687.

19. Brownlee M. Banting Lecture 2004: The pathobiology of diabetic complications: a unifying mechanism. *Diabetes.* 2005;54:1615–1625.

20. Kilpatrick ES, Rigby AS, Atkin SL. The effect of glucose variability on the risk of microvascular complications in type 1 diabetes. *Diabetes Care.* 2006;29:1486–1490.

21. Juvenile Diabetes Research Foundation Continuous Glucose Monitoring Study Group. Continuous glucose monitoring and intensive treatment of type 1 diabetes. *N Engl J Med.* 2008;259:1464–1476.

22. Tanenberg R, Bode B, Lane W, et al. Use of the continuous glucose monitoring system to guide therapy in patients with insulin-treated diabetes: a randomized controlled trial. *Mayo Clin Proc.* 2004;79:1521–1526.

23. Garg S, Zisser H, Schwartz S, et al. Improvement in glycemic excursions with a transcutaneous, real-time continuous glucose sensor: a randomized controlled trial. *Diabetes Care.* 2006;29:44–50.

24. American Diabetes Association. Standards of Medical Care in Diabetes—2009. *Diabetes Care.* 2009;32(Suppl 1):S13–61.

25. Funnel MM, Brown TL, Childs BP, et al. National standards for diabetes self-management education. *Diabetes Care.* 2009;32(Suppl 1):S87–S94.

26. Pastors JG, Warshaw H, Daly A, Franz M, Kulkarni K. The evidence for the effectiveness of medical nutrition therapy in diabetes management. *Diabetes Care.* 2002;25:608–613.

27. A position statement of the American Diabetes Association. Nutrition recommendations and interventions for diabetes. *Diabetes Care.* 2008;31(Suppl 1): S61–S78.

28. Diabetes Control and Complications Trial Research Group. The effect of intensive treatment of diabetes on the development and progression of long-term complications in insulin-dependent diabetes mellitus. *N Engl J Med.* 1993;329:977–986.

29. Hirsch IB. Insulin analogues. *N Engl J Med.* 2005;352:174–183.

30. Ratner RE, Hirsch IB, Neifing JL, et al. Less hypoglycemia with insulin glargine in intensive therapy for type 1 diabetes. *Diabetes Care.* 2000;23:639–643.

31. De Leeuw I, Vague P, Selam JL, et al. Insulin detemir used in basal-bolus therapy in people with type 1 diabetes is associated with a lower risk of nocturnal hypoglycaemia and less weight gain over 12 months in comparison to NPH insulin. *Diabetes Obes Metab.* 2005;7:73–82.

32. Anderson JH Jr, Brunelle RL, Koivisto VA, et al. Reduction of postprandial hyperglycemia and frequency of hypoglycemia in IDDM patients on insulin-analog treatment. *Diabetes.* 1997;46:265–270.

33. Heller SR, Colagiuri S, Vaaler S. Hypoglycaemia with insulin aspart: a double-blind, randomised, crossover trial in subjects with type 1 diabetes. *Diabetic Med.* 2004;21:769–775.

34. Heller SR, Amiel SA, Mansell P. Effect of the fast-acting insulin analog lispro on the risk of nocturnal hypoglycemia during intensified insulin therapy. *Diabetes Care.* 1999;22:1607–1611.

35. Plank J, Siebenhofer A, Berghold A, et al. Systematic review and meta-analysis of short-acting insulin analogues in patients with diabetes mellitus. *Arch Intern Med.* 2005;165:1337–1344.

36. Holleman F, Van den Brand JJG, Hoven RA, et al. Comparison of LysB28, ProB29-human insulin analog and regular human insulin in the correction of incidental hyperglycemia. *Diabetes Care.* 1996;19:1426–1429.

37. DeWitt DE, Hirsch IB. Outpatient insulin therapy in type 1 and type 2 diabetes mellitus. *JAMA.* 2003;289:2254–2264.

38. Mooradian AD, Bernbaum M, Albert SG. Narrative review: a rational approach to starting insulin therapy. *Ann Intern Med.* 2006;145:125–134.

39. Davidson PC, Hebblewhite HR, Steed RD, Bode BW. Analysis of guidelines for basal-bolus insulin dosing: basal insulin, correction factor, and carbohydrate-to-insulin ratio. *Endocr Pract.* 2008;14:1095–1101.

40. American Diabetes Association. Insulin administration. *Diabetes Care.* 2004;27(suppl 1):S106–109.

41. Colquitt J, Royle P, Waugh N. Are analogue insulins better than soluble in continuous subcutaneous insulin infusion? Results of a meta-analysis. *Diabet Med.* 2003;20:863–866.

42. Zinman B, Tildesley H, Chiasson JL, Tsui E, Strack T. Insulin lispro in CSII: results of a double-blind crossover study. *Diabetes.* 1997;46:440–443.

43. Bode B, Weinstein R, Bell D, et al. Comparison of insulin aspart with buffered regular insulin and insulin lispro in continuous subcutaneous insulin infusion: a randomized study in type 1 diabetes. *Diabetes Care.* 2002;25:439–444.

44. Bode BW, Sabbah HT, Gross TM, Fredrickson LP, Davidson PC. Diabetes management in the new millennium using insulin pump therapy. *Diabetes Metab Res Rev.* 2002;18(suppl 1):S14–20.

45. Pickup J, Mattock M, Kerry S. Glycaemic control with continuous subcutaneous insulin infusion compared with intensive insulin injections in patients with type 1 diabetes. *BMJ.* 2002;324:705.

46. Doyle EA, Weinzimer SA, Steffen AT, Ahern JA, Vincent M, Tamborlane WV. A randomized, prospective trial comparing the efficacy of continuous subcutaneous insulin infusion with multiple daily injections using insulin glargine. *Diabetes Care.* 2004;27:1554–1558.

47. Hirsch IB, Bode BW, Garg S, et al. Continuous subcutaneous insulin infusion (CSII) of insulin aspart versus multiple daily injections of insulin aspart/insulin glargine in type 1 diabetic patients previously untreated with CSII. *Diabetes Care.* 2005;28:533–538.

48. Fatourechi MM, Kudva YC, Murad MH, Elamin MB, Tabini CC, Montori VM. Hypoglycemia with intensive insulin therapy: a systematic review and meta-analyses of randomized trials of continuous subcutaneous insulin infusion versus multiple daily injections. *J Clin Endocrin Metab.* 2009;94:729–740.

49. Bolli GB, Kerr D, Thomas R, et al. Comparison of a multiple daily insulin injection regimen (basal once-daily glargine plus mealtime lispro) and continuous subcutaneous insulin infusion (lispro) in type 1 diabetes: a randomized open parallel multicenter study. *Diabetes Care.* 2009;32:1170–1176.

50. American Diabetes Association. Continuous subcutaneous insulin infusion. *Diabetes Care.* 2007; 27(Suppl 1):S110.

51. Singh-Franco D, Robles G, Gazze D. Pramlintide acetate injection for the treatment of type 1 and type 2 diabetes mellitus. *Clin Ther.* 2007;29:535–562.

52. Schmitz O, Brock B, Rungby J. Amylin agonists: a novel approach in the treatment of diabetes. *Diabetes.* 2004;53(suppl 3):S233–S238.

53. Hollander PA, Levy P, Fineman MS, et al. Pramlintide as an adjunct to insulin therapy improves long-term glycemic and weight control in patients with type 2 diabetes: a 1-year randomized controlled trial. *Diabetes Care.* 2003;26:784–790.

54. Franz MJ, Bantle JP, Beebe CA, et al. Evidence-based nutrition principles and recommendations for the treatment and prevention of diabetes and related complications. *Diabetes Care.* 2002;25:148–198.

55. American Diabetes Association. Physical activity/exercise and diabetes. *Diabetes Care.* 2004;27(suppl 1):S58–S62.

56. Toni S, Reali MF, Barni F, et al. Managing insulin therapy during exercise in type 1 diabetes mellitus. *Acta Biomed.* 2006;77(Suppl 1):34–40.

57. Wasserman DH, Zinman B. Exercise in individuals with IDDM. *Diabetes Care.* 1994;17:924–937.

58. Chadran M, Edelman SV. Have insulin, will fly; diabetes management during air travel and time zone adjustment strategies. *Clin Diabetes.* 2003;21(2):82–85.

59. Available at: http://www.tsa.gov/travelers/airtravel/specialneeds/editorial_1374.shtm#3. Accessed 10 Sept 2009.

Chapter 3

Complications

Type 1 diabetes is associated with long-term microvascular complications that affect the eyes, kidneys, and peripheral and autonomic nervous systems as well as macrovascular atherosclerotic disease, including cardiac, cerebral, and peripheral vascular disease.[1] These complications cause significant morbidity and mortality and can lead to a considerable decline in independence and quality of life. In this chapter, these complications and the serious problem of hypoglycemia are discussed. The acute metabolic complication DKA is discussed with inpatient management in Chapter 4.

Retinopathy and Nephropathy

Diabetic retinopathy is classified as nonproliferative retinopathy (NPDR), which may include microaneurysms and hemorrhages, hard exudates, and cotton-wool spots, or proliferative retinopathy (PDR), which includes neovascularization in response to retinal ischemia and may lead to hemorrhages and retinal detachment. Macular edema can occur at any stage and may cause vision loss.

Persistent albuminuria in the range of 30 to 299 mg/24 h (microalbuminuria) is the earliest stage of diabetic kidney disease and typically may appear beginning 5 years after type 1 diabetes is diagnosed. Microalbuminuria may regress with treatment, but it is associated with a greater risk of developing macroalbuminuria and kidney failure. Macroalbuminuria ($\geq$300 mg/24 h) is associated with a progressive decline in glomerular filtration rate, an increase in blood pressure, and a high risk of kidney failure. Patients who progress to macroalbuminuria are likely to progress to end-stage renal disease.[2,3]

The landmark Diabetes Control and Complications Trial (DCCT) demonstrated that much of the morbidity and mortality associated with insulin-dependent diabetes can be delayed or avoided with intensive insulin therapy.[4] Intensive insulin therapy, consisting of three or more daily doses of insulin delivered by injection or pump and adjusted according to the results of SMBG done at least four times a day with the goal of fasting glucose 70 to 120 mg/dL (3.9–6.7 mmol/L), postprandial glucose less than 180 mg/dL (10 mmol/L), and normal A1c (<6.05%), was compared to conventional therapy of one or two doses of insulin, including mixed intermediate and rapid-acting insulin; the median A1c levels achieved throughout the 9 years of the study were 7.2% and 9.1% respectively. The intensive therapy slowed the progression of retinopathy by 54%, reduced the development of proliferative or severe nonproliferative retinopathy by 47%, and reduced the occurrence of microalbuminuria by 39% and albuminuria by 54%. Intensive therapy was more effective when introduced during the first 5 years of diabetes as primary prevention than when introduced after complications had begun to develop.

The follow-up Epidemiology of Diabetes Interventions and Complications (EDIC) study found that, although the difference in median A1c between the groups narrowed during 4 years of follow-up to 7.9% and 8.2%, the patients who had received intensive therapy during the DCCT continued to have a significantly lower prevalence of retinopathy and macular edema and had a 76% lower rate of progression of retinopathy. The intensive therapy group also had a 53% lower risk of developing microalbuminuria and an 86% lower risk of developing albuminuria. Thus, the reduced risk of complications from the earlier intensive therapy persisted for at least 4 years despite rising A1c. In both groups, the likelihood of progressive retinopathy was strongly associated with the mean A1c value.[5]

In addition to optimizing glucose and blood pressure control, there are specific recommendations regarding retinopathy and nephropathy screening and treatment.[2]

For retinopathy:

- Patients should have an initial dilated and comprehensive eye examination by an ophthalmologist or optometrist within 5 years after the onset of type 1 diabetes. Examinations should be repeated annually.
- Patients with any degree of macular edema, severe NPDR, or any PDR should be referred to an ophthalmologist experienced in the management of diabetic retinopathy. Laser photocoagulation is indicated to reduce the risk of vision loss in many cases of diabetic retinopathy.
- Retinopathy is not a contraindication to aspirin therapy for cardioprotection since aspirin does not increase the risk of retinal hemorrhage.

For nephropathy:

- Urine albumin excretion (e.g., random spot urine microalbumin:creatinine ratio) should be assessed annually beginning 5 years after diagnosis. Positive tests should be repeated twice within 3 to 6 months; if at least two tests are positive, treatment should be started. Serum creatinine should also be measured at least annually and used to estimate glomerular filtration rate (GFR).
- Angiotensin-converting enzyme (ACE) inhibitors or angiotensin receptor blockers (ARBs) should be used to treat patients with micro- or macroalbuminuria. Studies have shown that ACE inhibitors delay the progression of nephropathy in patients with type 1 diabetes, hypertension, and any degree of albuminuria. Achievement of systolic blood pressure of below 140 mm Hg using ACE inhibitors provides a selective benefit over other antihypertensive drug classes in delaying the progression from micro- to macroalbuminuria and can slow the decline in GFR in patients with macroalbuminuria. There are no adequate head-to-head comparisons of ACE inhibitors to ARBs, but, since there is evidence that ARBs delay the progression of nephropathy in type 2 diabetes mellitus, both are recommended; if one class is not tolerated, the other should be used.
- Dietary protein restriction is recommended for patients with chronic kidney disease since it may improve measures of renal function.

Neuropathy

Diabetes is associated with a diverse array of neuropathies. The most common are chronic sensorimotor distal symmetric polyneuropathy (DPN) and the autonomic neuropathies. DPN symptoms may include burning pain, electrical or stabbing sensations, paresthesias, hyperesthesias, and deep aching pain, typically worse at night and involving the feet and lower limbs and occasionally the hands. Signs include sensory loss of vibration, pressure, pain, and temperature perception and absent ankle reflexes. DPN is a diagnosis of exclusion; neuropathy due to chronic inflammatory demyelinating polyneuropathy, B_{12} deficiency, hypothyroidism, uremia, and spinal stenosis, for example, should be ruled out. Screening for DPN is important since it is often asymptomatic and puts patients at risk for insensate foot injuries. Since more than 80% of amputations follow a foot ulcer or injury, early recognition, education, and treatment of at-risk patients may reduce the risk of ulcers and amputations.[6]

Autonomic neuropathy produces substantial morbidity and mortality. Cardiovascular autonomic neuropathy is suggested by resting tachycardia, exercise intolerance, and orthostatic hypotension and has been associated with sudden death and silent myocardial ischemia. Gastrointestinal autonomic neuropathy may cause abdominal pain, nausea, vomiting, bloating, diarrhea, constipation, and incontinence. Gastroparesis, by altering the absorption of meals, may make glycemic control difficult and unpredictable ("brittle diabetes"). Autonomic neuropathy may also involve sexual dysfunction, bladder dysfunction including urinary frequency, retention, and incontinence, and sudomotor or pupillary dysfunction.[6]

In the DCCT, intensive insulin therapy markedly delayed or prevented the development of diabetic polyneuropathy. Intensive therapy reduced the development of confirmed clinical neuropathy by 64% after 5 years of follow-up and reduced the prevalence of abnormal nerve conduction and abnormal autonomic nervous system function by 44% and 53% respectively. Nerve conduction velocities worsened in the conventional therapy group but remained stable in the intensive therapy group.[7]

In addition to achieving stable and optimal glycemic control, current recommendations regarding neuropathy include the following[2]:

- All patients should be screened for DPN at diagnosis and at least annually thereafter. Screening is accomplished using tests of pin-prick sensation, vibration perception (128-Hz tuning fork), 10-g monofilament pressure sensation, and ankle reflexes. Using more than one test has greater than 87% sensitivity for detecting DPN; loss of monofilament and vibration perception predicts foot ulcers.
- Screening for signs and symptoms of cardiovascular autonomic neuropathy should begin 5 years after diagnosis.
- Medications for the relief of neuropathy symptoms are recommended. These include tricyclic drugs (e.g., amitriptyline 10–75 mg HS) or anticonvulsants (e.g., gabapentin 300–1,200 mg tid or pregabalin 100 mg tid) for painful DPN symptoms and prokinetic agents (e.g., metoclopramide), antiemetics (e.g., phenergan), or bulking agents for gastrointestinal autonomic neuropathy.

Cardiovascular Disease

Any elevation in glycemia increases the risk of cardiovascular disease (CVD).[8] Type 1 diabetes is associated with at least a 10-fold increase in CVD compared with an age-matched nondiabetic population.[9,10] Fortunately, as with microvascular complications, intensive insulin therapy has been shown to reduce the risk of CVD. As part of the EDIC study, after a mean of 17 years of follow-up, having received intensive insulin treatment during the DCCT reduced the risk of any CVD event by 42% and the risk of nonfatal myocardial infarction, stroke, or death from cardiovascular disease by 57%.[11]

In addition to intensive insulin therapy, there are specific recommendations regarding comorbidities aimed at prevention of CVD[2]:

- Blood pressure should be measured at every visit and hypertension should be treated to below 130/80 mm Hg. If treatment is required, the regimen should include an ACE inhibitor or an ARB due to their demonstrated reduction of cardiovascular outcomes.

- Fasting lipid profiles should be measured annually. Statin therapy should be started in all diabetic patients with CVD and in those without CVD over age 40 with one or more other CVD risk factors. Statin therapy should be considered in other diabetics with LDL cholesterol exceeding 100 mg/dL or multiple CVD risk factors. The primary goal for dyslipidemia treatment is an LDL cholesterol level below 100 mg/dL; treatment to below 70 mg/dL is an optional goal for those with CVD. Secondary goals include triglycerides below 150 mg/dL and HDL cholesterol above 40 mg/dL in men and above 50 mg/dL in women.

- Aspirin therapy (71–162 mg/day) is recommended for primary prevention in those at increased cardiovascular risk, including those over 40 years old or with additional risk factors (family history of CVD, hypertension, smoking, dyslipidemia, or albuminuria), and for secondary prevention in all diabetics with CVD; clopidogrel should be used for those with CVD and documented aspirin allergy.

Incidence of Complications

The data from the DCCT/EDIC studies were recently analyzed to provide an estimate of anticipated outcomes of type 1 diabetes based on current treatment. After 30 years of type 1 diabetes, the cumulative incidences of proliferative retinopathy, nephropathy, and cardiovascular disease were 50%, 25%, and 14% in the DCCT conventional treatment group and 21%, 9%, and 9% in the intensive treatment group, with fewer than 1% becoming blind or requiring renal replacement or amputation. The authors suggest that the conventional group results provide an estimate of expected outcomes for patients who have had type 1 diabetes for much of the past 25 years, whereas the intensive group results indicate what patients might expect in the future given that intensive therapy is now the standard of care.[12] These figures are considerably better than those reported for these complications in the past.[1]

Hypoglycemia

Hypoglycemia is the most acute potential complication in type 1 diabetes and sometimes the most feared. Due to the brain's need for a continuous supply of glucose, hypoglycemia can be fatal: 2% to 4% of deaths in type 1 patients are attributed to hypoglycemia.[13] Patients attempting tight glycemic control have innumerable asymptomatic episodes of hypoglycemia and may have a blood glucose lower than 50 mg/dL up to 10% of the time; on average they have two episodes of symptomatic hypoglycemia per week and one episode of severe, at least temporarily disabling hypoglycemia, often with seizure or coma, per year.[14] Hypoglycemia often limits the achievement of sustained normoglycemia through intensive insulin therapy and thus interferes with attempts at preventing the long-term complications of diabetes.

All of the counterregulatory mechanisms that prevent hypoglycemia in nondiabetics are absent or defective in people with type 1 diabetes. In nondiabetics, insulin release is downregulated in the presence of hypoglycemia, but in diabetics the insulin is exogenous and cannot be downregulated once administered. Glucagon secretion in response to hypoglycemia is absent in type 1 diabetes, and the epinephrine response to hypoglycemia is attenuated and becomes more so with recurrent episodes of hypoglycemia.[15]

Hypoglycemia is defined as a blood glucose concentration of 70 mg/dL (3.9 mmol/L) or less, the level at which counterregulatory systems are triggered in nondiabetics. The clinical syndrome is characterized by Whipple's triad: symptoms consistent with hypoglycemia, a low measured blood glucose level, and resolution of the symptoms after the glucose level is raised. Hypoglycemia produces neurogenic or autonomic symptoms due to autonomic nervous system activation and neuroglycopenic symptoms due to brain glucose deprivation (Table 3.1). The latter symptoms occur at a lower glucose level, but the glycemic thresholds for developing both types of symptoms vary and depend on recent glucose levels; people with uncontrolled hyperglycemia may develop symptoms at glucose levels that are normal as their glycemic control improves ("relative hypoglycemia"), while people with recurrent hypoglycemia have lower thresholds, sometimes so low that they cannot perceive even dangerously low glucose levels ("hypoglycemic unawareness").[16]

Besides reducing the symptom threshold, hypoglycemic episodes can attenuate physiologic counterregulatory mechanisms to a degree proportional to the degree of the antecedent hypoglycemia.[17,18] The inability to recognize and recover from hypoglycemia can result in patients developing the most severe neuroglycopenic sequelae with little or no warning, sometimes with catastrophic results. Thus, strict glycemic targets may be dangerous in people with hypoglycemic

Table 3.1 Symptoms of Hypoglycemia

Autonomic Symptoms	Neuroglycopenic Symptoms
Tremors/shaking	Irritability
Hunger	Weakness
Sweating	Confusion/difficulty thinking
Anxiety/nervousness	Slurred speech
Palpitations	Behavioral changes
	Sleepiness
	Seizures
	Coma
	Death

unawareness. Since these effects are reversible with strict avoidance of hypogly-cemia, a temporary relaxation of glycemic control is recommended to restore hypoglycemic awareness.[2]

Exercise can provoke hypoglycemia in people with type 1 diabetes. Exercise increases the rate of insulin absorption from injection sites. Furthermore, the activation of the counterregulatory hormones, which would normally increase endogenous glucose production to match the increased glucose uptake by muscles, is reduced in type 1 diabetes.[19] See Chapter 2, p. 25, for strategies for preventing exercise-related hypoglycemia.

Older adults with type 1 diabetes are at particular risk for hypoglycemia for numerous reasons, including altered counterregulatory mechanisms, erratic nutrition, and comorbidities such as dementia, renal or hepatic insufficiency, and cerebrovascular disease, which can lead to treatment errors and delayed or decreased perception of hypoglycemic symptoms.[20,21]

SMBG frequency should be increased during potential times of hypoglycemia (e.g., during exercise or after a missed or unexpectedly small meal). Discussions with patients about hypoglycemia should include education about the time-action profiles of their insulins, the effects of alcohol, the risks of driving while hypogly-cemic, the importance of always having a quick source of glucose available, and the potentially life-saving benefit of wearing diabetes alert identification.

Hypoglycemia is best treated by ingestion of 15 to 20 g of pure glucose (e.g., 3 glucose tablets or 6 oz of juice). Any form of carbohydrate that contains glucose will raise blood glucose, but added fat (e.g., in peanut butter or choco-late) may retard the acute glycemic response. Fifteen minutes after treatment, the blood glucose should be rechecked; if it remains less than 70 mg/dL (3.9 mmol/L), additional glucose should be consumed. After recovery, additional food should be ingested to prevent recurrent hypoglycemia from ongoing insulin activity. Severe hypoglycemia, in which the person requires assistance and cannot be treated with oral glucose due to altered mental status, should be treated with 1 mg glucagon injected subcutaneously. Family members and close contacts of patients with type 1 diabetes should be instructed in the use of glucagon emergency kits, which are available by prescription.[2] Since glucagon works by promoting glycogenolysis, it may be ineffective if hepatic glucose stores are depleted (e.g., in starvation or chronic alcohol ingestion or after prolonged exercise). In the inpatient setting, severe hypoglycemia can be treated quickly with 25 g of 50% dextrose given intravenously.

The risk of severe hypoglycemia remains a barrier to the achievement of normoglycemia with intensive insulin therapy. Although severe hypoglycemia can be dangerous when it occurs, and prolonged profound hypoglycemia can cause permanent brain damage or death, it appears that recurrent severe episodes of hypoglycemia associated with intensive insulin therapy, including those associated with seizure or coma, have no long-term adverse cognitive effects. The better glycemic control from intensive insulin therapy may in fact produce subtle beneficial effects on cognitive function in addition to reducing the risk of retinopathy, nephropathy, neuropathy, and cardiovascular complications.[22,23]

References

1. Nathan DM. Long-term complications of diabetes mellitus. *N Engl J Med.* 1993;328:1676–1685.

2. American Diabetes Association. Standards of medical care in diabetes—2009. *Diabetes Care.* 2009;32(Suppl 1):S13–61.

3. National Kidney Foundation. KDOQI™ clinical practice guidelines and clinical practice recommendations for diabetes and chronic kidney disease. *Am J Kidney Dis.* 2007;49(suppl 2):S1–S180.

4. Diabetes Control and Complications Trial Research Group. The effect of intensive treatment of diabetes on the development and progression of long-term complications in insulin-dependent diabetes mellitus. *N Engl J Med.* 1993;329:977–986.

5. Diabetes Control and Complications Trial/Epidemiology of Diabetes Interventions and Complications Research Group. Retinopathy and nephropathy in patients with type 1 diabetes four years after a trial of intensive therapy. *N Engl J Med.* 2000;342:381–389.

6. Boulton AJM, Vinik AI, Arezzo JC, et al. Diabetic neuropathies. *Diabetes Care.* 2005;28:956–962.

7. Diabetes Control and Complications Trial Research Group. The effect of intensive diabetes therapy on the development and progression of neuropathy. *Ann Intern Med.* 1995;122:561–568.

8. Khaw KT, Wareham N, Bingham S, Luben R, Welch A, Day N. Association of hemoglobin A1c with cardiovascular disease and mortality in adults: the European Prospective Investigation into Cancer in Norfolk. *Ann Intern Med.* 2004;141:413–420.

9. Laing SP, Swerdlow AJ, Slater SD, et al. Mortality from heart disease in a cohort of 23,000 patients with insulin-treated diabetes. *Diabetologia.* 2003;46:760–765.

10. Dorman JS, LaPorte RE, Kuller LH, et al. The Pittsburgh insulin-dependent diabetes mellitus (IDDM) morbidity and mortality study: mortality results. *Diabetes.* 1984;33:271–276.

11. Diabetes Control and Complications Trial/Epidemiology of Diabetes Interventions and Complications (DCCT/EDIC) Study Research Group. Intensive diabetes treatment and cardiovascular disease in patients with type 1 diabetes. *N Engl J Med.* 2005;353:2643–2653.

12. Diabetes Control and Complications Trial/Epidemiology of Diabetes Interventions and Complications (DCCT/EDIC) Research Group. Modern-day clinical course of type 1 diabetes mellitus after 30 years' duration. *Arch Intern Med.* 2009;169(14):1307–1316.

13. Cryer PE. *Hypoglycemia Pathophysiology, Diagnosis and Treatment.* New York: Oxford University Press, 1997.

14. Cryer PE. Glucose homeostasis and hypoglycemia. In: Kronenberg HM, Melmed S, Polonsky KS, Larsen PR, eds. *Williams Textbook of Endocrinology, 11th ed.* Philadelphia: Saunders, 2008:1511.

15. Cryer PE. Diverse causes of hypoglycemia-associated autonomic failure in diabetes. *N Engl J Med.* 2004;350:2272–2279.

16. American Diabetes Association Workgroup on Hypoglycemia. Defining and reporting hypoglycemia in diabetes: a report from the American Diabetes Association Workgroup on Hypoglycemia. *Diabetes Care.* 2005;28:1245.

17. Heller SR, Cryer PE. Reduced neuroendocrine and symptomatic responses to subsequent hypoglycemia after 1 episode of hypoglycemia in nondiabetic humans. *Diabetes* 1991;4:223–226.

18. Davis SN, Shavers C, Mosqueda-Garcia R, et al. Effects of differing antecedent hypoglycemia on subsequent counterregulation in normal humans. *Diabetes.* 1997;46(8):1328–1335.

19. Schneider S, Vitug A, Ananthakrishnan R, et al. Impaired adrenergic response to prolonged exercise in type I diabetes. *Metabolism.* 1991;40:1219–1225.

20. Matyka K, Evans M, Lomas J, et al. Altered hierarchy of protective responses against severe hypoglycemia in normal aging in healthy men. *Diabetes Care.* 1997;20(2):135–141.

21. Shorr RI, Ray WA, Daugherty JR, et al. Incidence and risk factors for serious hypoglycemia in older persons using insulin or sulfonylureas. *Arch Intern Med.* 1997;157(15):1681–1686.

22. Diabetes Control and Complications Trial/Epidemiology of Diabetes Interventions and Complications (DCCT/EDIC) Study Research Group. Long-term effect of diabetes and its treatment on cognitive function. *N Engl J Med.* 2007;356:1842–1852.

23. Effects of intensive diabetes therapy on neuropsychological function in adults in the Diabetes Control and Complications Trial. *Ann Intern Med.* 1996; 124(4):379–388.

Chapter 4

Special Settings

Pregnancy

Type 1 diabetes and its effects on pregnancy, management, and potential complications is an important yet extensive topic, and a complete review is beyond the scope of this book. This section will highlight some of the major management principles and complications.

Prior to pregnancy, type 1 diabetics should achieve optimal glycemic control and obtain appropriate counseling. Counseling and education is paramount to improve control, to make patients understand potential risks and complications, and to review expectations required for management during pregnancy. As outlined in Chapter 2, all patients should receive diabetes self-management education and training (DSMT) and medical nutrition therapy (MNT) and ideally should be on basal/bolus insulin regimens, either through injections or CSII. Patients should be adept at carbohydrate counting and must be able to perform SMBG before and after meals; they should also be knowledgeable about ketone testing and treating hypoglycemia. Assessment of baseline acute and chronic diabetic complications is important prior to pregnancy, as certain microvascular complications may progress during pregnancy (Table 4.1).[1] Careful prepregnancy evaluation and education can help avoid risks to both mother and fetus, including congenital malformations, spontaneous abortion, and neonatal morbidity and mortality.

The American College of Gynecology (ACOG) and the American Diabetes Association have similar goals for glucose control. According to ACOG, fasting blood glucose values should be less than 95 mg/dL, 1-hour postprandial values should be less than 140 mg/dL, and the A1c goal is 6% or less.[2] Other authors propose stricter goals, recommending a fasting glucose range of 55 to 65 mg/dL and 1-hour postprandial values of less than 120 mg/dL, as there is evidence for even tighter glucose control from studies showing reductions in macrosomia.[3]

Patients should receive nutritional counseling or work with a registered dietitian to ensure adequate calories based on ideal body weight, yet they should avoid excess weight gain. For mealtime insulin, rapid-acting lispro and aspart appear to be safe in pregnancy. There are not enough data on glulisine use in pregnancy at this time.[4] For basal insulin, we recommend NPH insulin BID or TID. There is more data regarding its safety in pregnancy as opposed to the longer-acting analog insulins, glargine and detemir,[5] and doses are more easily adjusted with NPH insulin (for example, to correspond with increased basal requirements at different times of day).

Table 4.1 Preconception Care in Type 1 Diabetes: Laboratory Testing and Recommendations

	Preconception	During pregnancy
Glycemic control	A1c SMBG review Diabetes self-management training and nutritional counseling	A1c at 1- to 2-month intervals depending on level of control Review of SMBG
Nephropathy	Serum creatinine and glomerular filtration rate or creatinine clearance Urine microalbumin:creatinine ratio or 24-hour urine protein Blood pressure screening Nephrology evaluation and risk assessment if baseline disease detected	Reassessment of renal function each trimester Close nephrology follow-up for those with baseline disease
Retinopathy	Baseline fundoscopic examination Ophthalmology evaluation and risk assessment if baseline retinopathy detected	Reassessment each trimester for patients with baseline retinopathy
Neuropathy	Physical examination for signs and symptoms of peripheral/autonomic neuropathy	
Thyroid dysfunction	TSH/free T4 +/− Thyroid antibody testing Establish euthyroidism	Important to restore euthyroidism, particularly in early pregnancy; repeat testing q 4 weeks
Cardiovascular disease	Screening for those over age 35 or with comorbidities Possible prepregnancy intervention	Cardiology risk assessment and follow-up

Adapted from: American Diabetes Association. Preconception care of women with diabetes. *Diabetes Care.* 2003;26(Suppl 1):S91–S93.

The average insulin requirement in type 1 diabetic patients during pregnancy is approximately 0.7 to 0.8 units/kg during the first trimester to second trimester, with requirements often increasing to 0.9 to 1.0 units/kg for the remainder of the pregnancy, although each patient may have different needs; close monitoring is the key to dose adjustment.[6] Doses can be calculated with 50% of the total daily dose as NPH divided BID or TID, and 50% divided as mealtime insulin.

Patients on insulin pumps with excellent control before pregnancy can continue using their pumps throughout pregnancy with close monitoring and adjustments in requirements. Pregnant patients who are naïve to insulin pumps need extensive pump training and instruction prior to pump use; along with the changes associated with pregnancy and the need to maintain strict glycemic control, the switch to CSII may be overwhelming. Counseling on expectations, the need for pump management training, and potential costs must be provided prior to changing to CSII. Glycemic control can, however, be equally well achieved with MDI regimens, and no clear benefit of CSII over MDI during pregnancy has been found.[7] Women with poor glycemic control prior to pregnancy have higher rates of pregnancy complications, spontaneous abortion, and neonatal complications. Control is critical early in pregnancy, at the time of fetal organogenesis. Pregestational diabetes is associated with higher rates of macrosomia, congenital malformations, cesarean delivery, preterm delivery, pre-eclampsia, neonatal jaundice, respiratory distress syndrome, and perinatal mortality.[8] Normalizing blood glucose concentrations has been shown to reduce the risk of congenital malformations, spontaneous abortions, and macrosomia.[9,10]

DKA is associated with a high fetal mortality rate, and prompt recognition is necessary. Urinary ketones should be measured in pregnant patients who are experiencing hyperglycemia (>180 mg/dL) or illness.

There is also the potential for worsening microvascular complications, particularly among women with pre-existing or baseline retinopathy and nephropathy prior to pregnancy.[11] All women planning pregnancy should get a baseline retinal examination and renal evaluation (Table 4.1). Pre-existing neuropathy does not seem to worsen, but it can increase the risk of other complications, such as hypoglycemia unawareness.[12]

The risk of offspring of type 1 parents developing type 1 diabetes was mentioned briefly in the prediction section of Chapter 1. The child of a father with type 1 has a 1 in 17 chance of developing the disease. If the mother has type 1, the risk is 1 in 25; however, the risk to the child is only 1 in 100 if the mother developed diabetes at an older age.[13] As illustrated by the higher risk in children of diabetic fathers, it does not appear that the presence of maternal islet antibodies or cord blood islet antibodies in infants of diabetic mothers is predictive of subsequent development of islet autoimmunity.[14]

Inpatient Management

General Principles

Type 1 patients who are critically ill are best treated using a continuous intravenous insulin infusion. Otherwise, the general principles of inpatient treatment are the same as those of outpatient treatment: intensive insulin therapy comprising basal, prandial or nutritional, and supplemental or correction components.

Basal

Patients should generally be continued on the same basal insulin dose that they were taking as an outpatient. Patients who are not eating can be given their usual basal insulin or started on an insulin drip.

Prandial

Patients who are eating may require adjustments to their prandial insulin. If they are eating less than usual, the dose should be reduced. However, many hospitalized patients are under significant metabolic stress due to glucocorticoid treatment, infection, etc., and may need higher doses of prandial insulin despite eating less.[15] Rapid-acting analogs should be used due to their better postprandial glucose control and the difficulty of coordinating meal delivery with regular insulin's ideal administration time of 30 minutes before the meal. If the dietary intake is uncertain, dosing should be conservative and/or the dose should be given immediately after the meal in proportion to what was eaten rather than immediately before the meal as usual.[16]

Correction

For most patients, a low-dose correction insulin scale is appropriate: for example, 1 unit for a glucose level above 150 mg/dL (>8.3 mmol/L), 2 units for a level above 200 mg/dL (>11.1 mmol/L), 3 units for a level above 250 mg/dL (>13.9 mmol/L), etc. Given recent recommendations (see p. 46), for many patients it would be appropriate to begin the correction insulin scale at a value above 180 mg/dL (>10.0 mmol/L).

Ongoing monitoring of the response to treatment should guide further dose adjustments, which should take into account various factors that affect glucose levels in inpatients, including any mistiming of glucose measurement, meal intake, or insulin administration. Each component of the regimen (basal, prandial, and correction) should be adjusted every 1 to 2 days if the response is inadequate and immediately upon any change in nutritional status. Aggressiveness should also be guided by practical factors, such as the severity of illness and the patient's ability to perceive hypoglycemia.[16]

Patients with type 1 diabetes must always be given insulin to prevent ketosis. They should never be treated with "sliding-scale" insulin as the only insulin therapy. Even if they are not eating, their basal insulin must be given. When making the transition from intravenous to subcutaneous insulin, the intravenous insulin must be continued long enough after the first subcutaneous dose is given to ensure continuous insulin activity.

Glycemic Targets

The optimal glycemic targets for inpatient diabetes treatment are not clear. Several recent studies have attempted to clarify this issue with inconsistent results. These studies have recently been summarized with recommendations in a joint consensus statement from the American Diabetes Association and the American Association of Clinical Endocrinologists.[17] In short, some studies have demonstrated decreased morbidity and mortality from intensive treatment targeting near-euglycemia, particularly in surgical intensive care patients.[18–20] In general, however, there has been no consistent reduction in mortality, and this near-normal target has not been met without significantly increasing the incidence of severe hypoglycemia; in the largest trial to date, increased mortality was observed in the intensive treatment group.[21] Nevertheless, in a large number of studies in a variety of inpatient settings, uncontrolled hyperglycemia was clearly associated with poor outcomes. Therefore, a moderate target glucose range of 140 to 180 mg/dL (7.8 to 10.0 mmol/L) is recommended for most critically ill diabetic patients, preferably using intravenous insulin infusion with frequent glucose monitoring according to a validated insulin infusion protocol. For most patients who are not critically ill, the premeal glucose level should be less than 140 mg/dL (<7.8 mmol/L), with random glucose values below 180 mg/dL (10.0 mmol/L); lower targets may be appropriate in stable patients with previous tight glycemic control.

Insulin Pumps

Patients who use CSII are often well versed in diabetes self-management and may be reluctant to surrender their diabetes management to hospital staff when they are hospitalized. Often, such patients should be permitted to continue self-management with their insulin pumps. However, there are certain situations when self-management is inappropriate, including impaired consciousness, critical illness, or suicidal ideation.[22] Patients using CSII will generally need to provide all of their insulin pump supplies, and nursing staff should document basal rates and bolus doses regularly. It is unclear whether continuing CSII during hospitalization in appropriate patients offers any therapeutic advantage over switching such patients to multiple injection therapy, although it does appear to be safe.[22]

DKA

DKA is the most serious acute metabolic complication of type 1 diabetes. In DKA, inadequate insulin levels combined with elevated counterregulatory hormones (glucagon, cortisol, catecholamines, and growth hormone) lead to increased gluconeogenesis and glycogenolysis, impaired glucose uptake in peripheral tissues, and lipolysis, leading to hyperglycemia and fatty acid oxidation to ketone bodies (β-hydroxybutyrate and acetoacetate). The ketonemia leads to ketoacidosis, and the hyperglycemia leads to glycosuria, which in turn leads to osmotic diuresis and loss of water, sodium, potassium, and other electrolytes.[23]

Common precipitating factors of DKA are listed in Table 4.2, and typical presenting symptoms and signs are listed in Table 4.3.

The initial workup of a patient with suspected DKA should include plasma glucose, blood urea nitrogen, creatinine, serum ketones (preferably β-hydroxybutyrate), electrolytes, calculated anion gap, urine ketones, arterial blood gas, and complete blood count with differential. Additional tests such as a chest x-ray, cultures, or electrocardiogram should be ordered as needed to ascertain the cause of DKA. The diagnostic criteria and severity classification of DKA are shown in Table 4.4.

Patients with DKA may be normothermic or even hypothermic despite an infection; conversely, the leukocyte count may be elevated with or without infection. Serum amylase and lipase levels, which can be elevated without pancreatitis, can also be misleading.

Table 4.2 Common Precipitating Factors of DKA

Infection (e.g., urinary tract infection, pneumonia)
Inadequate insulin administration or treatment errors
Pancreatitis
Myocardial infarction
Stroke
Drugs (e.g., corticosteroids, second-generation antipsychotics)
Psychological issues
Trauma
Alcohol or drug abuse (e.g., cocaine)
Pregnancy

Table 4.3 Symptoms and Signs of DKA

Symptoms	Signs
Polyuria	Dehydration
Polydipsia	Poor skin turgor
Blurred vision	Tachycardia
Weight loss	Hypotension
Vomiting	Lethargy
Abdominal pain	Coma
Weakness	Kussmaul respiration
Confusion	

Table 4.4 Diagnostic Criteria of DKA[23]

Diagnostic criteria and classification	Mild DKA	Moderate DKA	Severe DKA
Plasma glucose (mg/dL)	>250	>250	>250
Arterial pH	7.25–7.30	7.00 to <7.25	<7.00
Serum bicarbonate (mEq/L)	15–18	10 to <15	<10
Urine ketone	Positive	Positive	Positive
Serum ketone	Positive	Positive	Positive
Anion gap	>10	>12	>12
Mental status	Alert	Alert/drowsy	Stupor/coma

Treatment of DKA involves correcting fluid deficits, hyperglycemia, and electrolyte imbalances and treating the precipitating cause as needed:

• Fluid resuscitation is the first priority; patients often have a water deficit of several liters. Isotonic (0.9%) saline is generally given first, typically 1 L over 1 hour and then at 250 to 500 mL/h until the patient is hemodynamically stable and hydrated. Half-normal (0.45%) saline can then be used at a lower rate with the goal of replacing the fluid deficit within 24 hours. Five percent dextrose should be added to the fluid when the serum glucose level is below 200 mg/dL.

- Insulin is given as an intravenous infusion of regular insulin, typically started with a 0.1-unit/kg bolus and then a 0.1-unit/kg/h infusion. The infusion rate is then adjusted hourly based on laboratory or fingerstick glucose results to achieve a 50- to 75-mg/dL decline in the serum glucose level to a target range of 150 to 200 mg/dL. If the glucose does not fall by that amount, the infusion rate should be doubled. If the glucose falls faster than that amount, the insulin can be held for 15 minutes and then restarted at a lower rate.

- Electrolytes should be measured every 2 hours. A potassium deficit of 3 to 5 mEq/kg is typical. Since insulin therapy, correction of acidosis, and volume repletion all decrease the plasma potassium concentration, potassium must be added to the fluid even when the serum level is normal. If the serum potassium is below 3.3 mEq/L, insulin should be held until the potassium rises above that threshold. Once the serum potassium is 4 to 5 mEq/L, adding 20 to 30 mEq potassium to each liter of fluid will maintain the potassium level in that range. Other electrolyte deficiencies are common and should be repleted if severe.

- Bicarbonate treatment is recommended only if the arterial pH is below 7.0.

The insulin infusion should be continued until ketonemia has resolved. Criteria for resolution of DKA include glucose less than 200 mg/dL, serum bicarbonate 18 mEq/L or higher, and venous pH greater than 7.3. When the patient is able to eat, a subcutaneous insulin regimen can be started and the intravenous insulin infusion can be discontinued 1 to 2 hours later; the overlap ensures adequate plasma insulin levels. Patient education may prevent subsequent episodes of DKA.[23]

Psychology (Depression and Eating Disorders)

Type 1 diabetes requires a significant amount of self-management, and psychological and social issues can impede a patient's ability to perform the tasks necessary for optimal treatment. Patients' attitudes toward their illness, expectations about outcomes, quality of life, and financial and social resources can all affect the implementation of successful treatment. Studies have demonstrated a higher incidence of depression in people with type 1 diabetes compared with the general population; low levels of education and physical impairment may increase the risk of depression.[24] Depression has been linked to reduced adherence to dietary and treatment recommendations, functional impairment, and higher health care costs.[25] Coexisting eating disorders present a particular challenge due to the risk of hyper- or hypoglycemia, depending on the patient's behaviors. In young patients, psychological problems complicated by eating disorders may be a contributing factor in 20% of cases of recurrent DKA.[26] Fear of weight gain from improved glycemic control, fear of hypoglycemia, or rebellion toward authority may motivate patients not to take their insulin doses.

A multidisciplinary team ideally including an endocrinologist/diabetologist, a nurse, a registered dietitian, a psychologist or social worker, and possibly a psychiatrist is needed to treat eating disorders in type 1 diabetic patients. At first, the primary medical goals are safety and the prevention of DKA; as rapport improves and treatment progresses, small, incremental goals can be set to move towards the usual management of type 1 diabetes.[27] Patients who are medically or psychiatrically unstable require inpatient treatment under close supervision, again with a multidisciplinary team. Once patients are more stable, they are encouraged to establish a regular eating pattern with a prescribed meal plan, and diabetes self-management behaviors are introduced. Glucose and glucagon must be readily available in case of refused meals or purging after prandial insulin is administered.[28]

Psychological and social situation assessment should be included in the ongoing medical management of all type 1 patients. When adherence is poor, patients should be screened for psychosocial problems such as depression, anxiety, and eating disorders.[29]

References

1. American Diabetes Association. Preconception care of women with diabetes. *Diabetes Care.* 2003;26(Suppl 1):S91–S93.

2. ACOG Practice Bulletin #60: Pregestational diabetes mellitus. *Obstet Gynecol.* 2005;105:675–685.

3. Jovanovic L. Druzin M, Peteron CM. Effect of euglycemia on the outcome of pregnancy in insulin-dependent diabetic women as compared with normal control subjects. *Am J Med.* 1981;71:921–927.

4. Metzger BE, Buchanan TA, Coustan DR, et al. Summary and recommendations of the fifth international workshop-conference on gestational diabetes mellitus. *Diabetes Care.* 2007;30(Suppl 2):S51–S60.

5. Jovanovic L, Pettitt DJ. Treatment with insulin and its analogs in pregnancies complicated by diabetes. *Diabetes Care.* 2007;30(Suppl 2):S220–S224.

6. Steel JM, Johnstone FD, Hume R, Mao JH. Insulin requirements during pregnancy in women with type 1 diabetes. *Obstet Gynecol.* 1994;83:253–258.

7. Mukhopadhyay A, Farrell T, Fraser RB, et al. Continuous subcutaneous insulin infusion vs. intensive conventional insulin therapy in pregnant diabetic women: a systematic review and metaanalysis of randomized, controlled trials. *Am J Obstet Gynecol.* 2007;197:447–456.

8. Jensen DM, Damm P, Moelsted-Pederon L, et al. Outcomes in type 1 diabetic pregnancies; a nationwide, population-based study. *Diabetes Care.* 2004;27:2819–2823.

9. Kitzmiller JL, Gavin LA, Gin GD, et al. Preconception care of diabetes: glycemic control prevents congenital abnormalities. *JAMA.* 1991;265(6):731–736.

10. Diabetes Control and Complications Trial Research Group. Pregnancy outcomes in the diabetes control and complications trial. *Am J Obstet Gynecol.* 1996;174:1343–1353.

11. Star J, Carpenter MW. The effect of pregnancy on the natural history of diabetic retinopathy and nephropathy. *Clin Perinatol.* 1998;25:887–916.

12. Mabie WC. Peripheral neuropathies during pregnancy. *Clin Obstet Gynecol.* 2005;48:57–66.

13. The Genetics of Diabetes. Available at: www. Diabetes.org/genetics.jsp. Accessed 10 Sept 2009.

14. Ziegler AG, Hummel M, Schenker M, Bonifacio E. Autoantibody appearance and risk for development of childhood diabetes in offspring of parents with type 1 diabetes: the 2-year analysis of the German BABYDIAB study. *Diabetes.* 1999;48:460–468.

15. Moghissi ES, Hirsch IB. Hospital management of diabetes. *Endocrinol Metab Clin North Am.* 2005;34:99–116.

16. Inzucchi SE. Management of hyperglycemia in the hospital setting. *N Engl J Med.* 2006;355:1903–1911.

17. Moghissi ES, Korytkowski MT, DiNardo M, et al. American Association of Clinical Endocrinologists and American Diabetes Association consensus statement on inpatient glycemic control. *Diabetes Care.* 2009;32:1119–1131.

18. Furnary AP, Zerr KJ, Grunkemeier GL, et al. Continuous intravenous insulin infusion reduces the incidence of deep sternal wound infection in diabetic patients after cardiac surgical procedures. *Ann Thorac Surg.* 1999;67:352–362.

19. Furnary AP, Gao G, Grunkemeier GL, et al. Continuous insulin infusion reduces mortality in patients with diabetes undergoing coronary artery bypass grafting. *J Thorac Cardiovasc Surg.* 2003;125:1007–1021.

20. Van den Berghe G, Wouters P, Weekers F, et al. Intensive insulin therapy in critically ill patients. *N Engl J Med.* 2001;345:1359–1367.

21. Finfer S, Chittock DR, Su SY, et al. Intensive versus conventional glucose control in critically ill patients. *N Engl J Med.* 2009;360:1283–1297.

22. Bailon RM, Partlow BJ, Miller-Cage V, et al. Continuous subcutaneous insulin infusion (insulin pump) therapy can be safely used in the hospital in selected patients. *Endocr Pract.* 2009;15:24–29.

23. Kitabchi AE, Umpierrez GE, Murphy MB, Kreisberg R. Hyperglycemic crises in adult patients with diabetes. *Diabetes Care.* 2006;29:2739–2748.

24. Engum A, Mykletun A, Midthjell K, Holen A, Dahl AA. Depression and diabetes. *Diabetes Care.* 2005;28:1904–1909.

25. Ciechanowski PS, Katon WJ, Russo JE. Depression and diabetes: impact of depressive symptoms on adherence, function, and costs. *Arch Intern Med.* 2000;160:3278–3285.

26. Polonsky WH, Anderson BJ, Lohrer PA, Aponte JE, Jacobson AM, Cole CF. Insulin omission in women with IDDM. *Diabetes Care.* 1994;17:1178–1185.

27. Goebel-Fabbri AE, Uplinger N, Gerken S, Mangham D, Criego A, Parkin C. Outpatient management of eating disorders in type 1 diabetes. *Diabetes Spectrum.* 2009;22:147–152.

28. Bermudez O, Gallivan H, Jahraus J, Lesser J, Meier M, Parkin C. Inpatient management of eating disorders in type 1 diabetes. *Diabetes Spectrum.* 2009;22:153–158.

29. American Diabetes Association. Standards of medical care in diabetes—2009. *Diabetes Care.* 2009;32(Suppl 1):S13–161.

Chapter 5

Future Therapies

Prevention

There has been tremendous progress in the field of type 1 diabetes prevention. The majority of prevention trials are focused on administering agents that can preserve beta cells, by slowing or halting the autoimmune destruction. Newly diagnosed type 1 diabetics may have some residual beta-cell function and may even go into a honeymoon period with low insulin requirements or even insulin independence, and LADA patients typically have a time period from diagnosis to dependence on insulin. This stage offers an opportunity to conserve the remaining beta-cell mass. Clinical trials of antigen-specific therapies and nonspecific immunomodulatory therapies have shown that we may be able to preserve islet function after recent onset of disease. Studies are also being performed on patients who are at high risk (antibody-positive) but have not yet developed clinical diabetes.

Older studies theorized that the use of insulin, supplements, or certain immunosuppressive agents could offer primary prevention of type 1 diabetes. Insulin administration was postulated to delay the development of type 1 diabetes as it may provide the remaining beta cells a rest period and may decrease their expression of autoantigens. The Diabetes Prevention Trial assigned high-risk patients (siblings of type 1 diabetes patients with elevated islet cell antibodies) to observation versus low-dose subcutaneous insulin with intermittent insulin infusions. Unfortunately the incidence of diabetes was similar between the two groups at follow-up (3.7 years).[1]

The immunosuppressive agents cyclosporine and azathioprine have been evaluated in patients with recently diagnosed type 1 diabetes, and while some studies show that endogenous insulin secretion may improve and insulin requirements decrease, neither agent prevented dependence on insulin or resulted in complete remission.[2,3] Nicotinamide was believed to be protective of beta cells, but unfortunately in a large randomized trial it did not seem to be effective in preventing the onset of type 1 diabetes in patients with a family history of type 1 diabetes and positive autoantibodies.[4] Administration of a vaccine containing the major autoantigen GAD 65 seems to preserve residual insulin secretion in patients with recent-onset type 1 diabetes, but it did not change insulin requirement at 30 months of follow-up compared to placebo.[5]

Administration of anti-CD3 antibodies may alter the dynamics of regulatory T cells, thus protecting the remaining beta cells from autoimmune attack. Administration of anti-CD3 monoclonal antibodies via infusion at the onset of type 1 may preserve beta-cell function in the short term versus those administered placebo.[6] Antithymocyte globulin and rituximab (anti-CD20 monoclonal antibody) are also being studied, as well as anti-IL2 receptor antibody, which may destroy activated T cells. Etanercept, a recombinant TNF-alpha receptor fusion protein, may block cytokine-mediated destruction of beta cells and has been shown to reduce insulin requirement and lower A1C values in youths newly diagnosed with type 1 diabetes compared to placebo.[7]

Other potential preventive strategies, such as eliminating exposure to potential environmental agents (such as cow's milk) and possible supplementation with agents (omega-3 fatty acids) that may prevent an autoimmune response are in development. It is important to offer newly diagnosed patients and high-risk patients the opportunity to participate in ongoing prevention trials (see Chapter 6). The exact combination of effective therapies, immunomodulatory or immunosuppressive, their dosage, and the best timing of administration remains to be studied and of course needs to be weighed against side-effect profiles and risk.

Pancreas and Islet Transplantation

Only selected patients should be considered for pancreas or islet cell transplantation, given that there are still limitations to these procedures and associated risks. Those with severe recurrent hypoglycemia and hypoglycemia unawareness, labile glucose values despite optimal medical therapies, unacceptable quality of life, and severe end-stage complications (such as end-stage renal disease) and those with psychiatric or emotional disability that prevents them from administering appropriate insulin therapies are candidates. This latter group presents a challenge, as such patients must be evaluated for their ability to handle immunosuppressive regimens and must maintain appropriate follow-up transplant care.

There are more potential surgical complications and complications related to immunosuppressive regimens with pancreas transplant, but longer-term reversal of diabetes is seen in comparison to islet transplantation.[8] Pancreas transplant may be done alone (PTA, pancreas transplant alone), after kidney transplant (PAK, pancreas after kidney transplant), or simultaneously with a kidney transplant (SPK), the latter being the most common procedure. SPK should be considered in those with imminent or established end-stage renal disease and in those who have had or plan to have kidney transplantation, as a pancreas transplant may improve kidney survival, and pancreas graft survival is better when done simultaneously with a kidney transplant.[9]

Pancreas survival rates are 88% to 92% at 1 year and 45% to 70% at 5 years.[10] The most common cause of organ failure is technical failure of the transplant. A pancreas transplant restores alpha-cell function and glucagon presence, which is likely the reason for the lack of hypoglycemia seen after a pancreas transplant.

The insulin response tends to be normal or can be exaggerated (measured as a first-phase response to intravenous glucose)[11] as the transplanted pancreas releases its hormones into the systemic venous circulation. This is opposed to the native pancreas, which releases insulin into the portal circulation, with a first-pass effect through the liver. There is evidence for improvements in nephropathy,[12] neuropathy,[13] retinopathy,[14] and quality of life[15] after pancreas transplantation.

The field of islet-cell transplantation does offer promise, particularly with corticosteroid-free protocols.[16] Islet-cell transplantation is typically done by harvesting donor islets and transplanting them through percutaneous portal vein cannulation. Potential complications immediately after the transplant are bleeding, thrombus, and elevated transaminases,[17] and immunosuppressive agents still carry a risk of toxicity and side effects. In a review of patients 5 years after islet transplant with the Edmonton protocol, the graft survival rate was approximately 80% (patients with measurable positive C-peptide); however, insulin independence at 5 years was only 10%. Grafts may not implant and may not survive or function optimally. Problems with graft survival may be related to toxicity from immunosuppression, the unnatural location of grafts (in the liver), the delivery of blood supply to the islets, and the possibility of recurrent autoimmune attack on the beta cells.[17] It is also difficult to assess the benefit of islet transplantation on microvascular complications of diabetes, as transplants are performed on longstanding diabetics with established complications and labile control. There are no data on transplants performed early in the course of diabetes prior to the development of complications.[9] In comparison to pancreas transplant, the glucagon response to hypoglycemia does not seem to be restored with islet-cell transplant. This may have to do with the hepatic location of the transplanted islet cells.[16] However, the restoration of some endogenous insulin does seem to provide better glucose control and less glycemic variability. Acute diabetic complications (hypoglycemia, ketoacidosis) and quality of life do improve after islet-cell transplantation.[9]

A major limitation to islet transplant is the lack of sufficient islet cells from donors. Typically, islet cells are combined from two donors, and patients undergo two transplants (two islet infusions) to attain insulin independence. Although this field is progressing, work needs to occur on procuring enough islet cells and optimizing their survival. Expansion of existing islet cells, xenografts, and embryonic stem cells are all potential sources.[16] Stem cells may be able to provide a bountiful source of islet cells, and this is an exciting area for future research.

As both fields progress, we accumulate more knowledge about the replacement of beta cells. We assume that any method that can produce functional islet cells to maintain glucose control will benefit patients in terms of quality of life and a reduction in the chronic complications of diabetes.

References

1. Diabetes Prevention Trial-Type 1 Diabetes Study Group. Effects of insulin in relatives of patients with type 1 diabetes mellitus. *N Engl J Med.* 2002; 346(22):1685–1691.

2. Cook, JJ, Hudson I, Harrison LC, et al. A double-blinded controlled trial of azathioprine in children with newly-diagnosed type 1 diabetes. *Diabetes.* 1989;38(6): 779–783.

3. Bougneres PF, Landais P, Boisson C, et al. Limited duration of remission of insulin dependency in children with recent overt type 1 diabetes treated with low-dose cyclosporine. *Diabetes.* 1990;39(10):1264–1272.

4. Gale EA, Bingley PJ, Emmett CL, Collier T. European Nicotinamide Diabetes Intervention Trial (ENDIT): a randomised control trial of intervention before the onset of type 1 diabetes. *Lancet.* 2004;363:925–931.

5. Ludvigsson J, Faresjo M, Hjorth M, et al. GAD treatment and insulin secretion in recent-onset type 1 diabetes. *N Engl J Med.* 2008;359(18):1909–1920.

6. Keymeulen B, Vandemeulebruke E, Ziegler AE, et al. Insulin needs after CD3-antibody therapy in new-onset type 1 diabetes. *N Engl J Med.* 2005;352: 2598–2608.

7. Mastrandrea L, Albini C, Yu J, et al. Etanercept treatment in children with new-onset type 1 diabetes. *Diabetes Care.* 2009;32(7):1244–1249.

8. Eisenbarth GS. Update in type 1 diabetes. *J Clin Endocrinol Metab.* 2007;92(7): 2403–2407.

9. American Diabetes Association Position Statement. Pancreas and islet transplantation in type 1 diabetes. *Diabetes Care.* 2006;29(4):935.

10. Cecka JM, Terasaki PI, eds. *Clinical Transplants,* Vol. 18. Los Angeles: UCLA Immunogenetics Center, 2002:43–52.

11. Diem P, Abid M, Redmon JB, et al. Systemic venous drainage of pancreas allografts as independent cause of hyperinsulinemia in type I diabetic recipients. *Diabetes.* 1990;39:534–540.

12. Fioretto P, Steffes MW, Sutherland DE, et al. Reversal of lesions of diabetic nephropathy after pancreas transplantation. *N Engl J Med.* 1998;339:69–75.

13. Navarro X, Kennedy WR, Loewenson RB, et al. Influence of pancreas transplantation on cardiorespiratory reflexes, nerve conduction, and mortality in diabetes mellitus. *Diabetes.* 1990;39:802–806.

14. Koznarova R, Saudek F, Sosna T, et al. Beneficial effect of pancreas and kidney transplantation on advanced diabetic retinopathy. *Cell Transplant.* 2000;9: 903–908.

15. Piehlmeier W, Bullinger M, Nusser J, et al. Quality of life in type 1 (insulin-dependent) diabetic patients prior to and after pancreas and kidney transplantation in relation to organ function. *Diabetologia.* 1991;34(Suppl 1):S150–S157.

16. Robertson RP. Islet transplantation as a treatment for diabetes: a work in progress. *N Engl J Med.* 2004;350(7):694–705.

17. Ryan EA, Paty BW, Senior PA, et al. Five-year follow-up after clinical islet transplantation. *Diabetes.* 2005;54:2060–2069.

Chapter 6

Provider and Patient Resources

Table 6.1 Medications Approved for Use in Treating Type 1 Diabetes		
Insulin Preparations Recommended:		
Rapid-acting/mealtime and correction insulin	Analog insulin	Lispro (Humalog) Aspart (Novolog) Apidra (Glulisine)
Long-acting/basal insulin	Analog insulin	Glargine (Lantus) Detemir (Levemir)
	Human insulin	NPH* (Neutral Protamine Hagedorn)
Amylin analog	Pramlintide (Symlin)	
*Suggested in pregnancy; see Chapter 4, p. 43.		

Diabetes Supplies

The American Diabetes Association publication *Diabetes Forecast* publishes a resource guide, includes a section on insulin delivery, and reviews available diabetes devices, including syringes, insulin pens, insulin pumps, injection tools, and aids for people who are visually or physically impaired. Available at: http://www.diabetes.org/diabetes-forecast/resource-guide.jsp

Insulin Pumps

Minimed Paradigm (Medtronic Diabetes)
http://www.minimed.com/
Animas, One Touch Ping (Animas, Johnson & Johnson)
http://www.animascorp.com/
Omnipod (Insulet)
http://www.myomnipod.com/
Accu-Chek Spirit (Diesetronic)
http://www.disetronic-usa.com/dstrnc_us/
DANA Diabecare IISG Insulin Pump (Sooil USA)
http://www.sooilusa.com/

Deltec Cozmo (Deltec): Manufacturing was discontinued in 2009. The company will honor current pump warranties and will provide ongoing customer and clinical support and ensures the availability of Cozmo pump supplies to all current Cozmo users throughout the remainder of current pump warranties. Patients should choose a new pump from another manufacturer once the warranty period is close to expiration.
http://www.cozmore.com/

Continuous Glucose Monitoring

Guardian, Paradigm REAL-Time Systems (Medtronic Diabetes)
http://www.minimed.com/
SEVEN Plus (DexCom)
http://www.dexcom.com/
Freestyle Navigator (Abbott Diabetes Care)
http://www.freestylenavigator.com/

Information on Type 1 Diabetes, Patient Education Materials, Diabetes Facts, and Publications

National Diabetes Education Program 1 Diabetes Way Bethesda, MD 20814–9692 Phone: 1–888–693–NDEP (6337) TTY: 1–866–569–1162 Fax: 703–738–4929 Email: ndep@mail.nih.gov Internet: www.ndep.nih.gov

American Diabetes Association 1701 North Beauregard Street Alexandria, VA 22311 Phone: 1–800–DIABETES (342–2383) Email: AskADA@diabetes.org Internet: www.diabetes.org

Juvenile Diabetes Research Foundation International 120 Wall Street New York, NY 10005 Phone: 1–800–533–CURE (2873) Fax: 212–785–9595 Email: info@jdrf.org Internet: www.jdrf.org

Finding a Diabetes Educator

American Association of Diabetes Educators, available at:
http://www.diabeteseducator.org/DiabetesEducation/Find.html

Clinical Trials

Type 1 Diabetes TrialNet: information on diabetes intervention studies testing treatments to delay or prevent the onset of type 1 diabetes, or treatments to preserve remaining insulin secretion in people recently diagnosed with type 1 diabetes; available at:
http://www.diabetestrialnet.org/index.htm

Index

Notes

CPSIA information can be obtained at www.ICGtesting.com
Printed in the USA
BVOW031017140812

297848BV00015B/1/P